GASTROPARESIS DIET COOKBOOK FOR WOMEN

THE COMPLETE LOW FIBER, LOW SODIUM, AND LOW SUGAR RECIPE GUIDE TO MANAGE DIABETICS AND ABDOMINAL PAIN

DREW DORSEY

COPYRIGHT © 2024 DREW DORSEY

CONTENTS

WELCOME!

For the Women Who Crave More: Reclaim Your Kitchen with Gastroparesis-Friendly Feasts

Imagine… the aroma of sizzling vegetables and herbs filling your kitchen. The anticipation of a delicious meal, the kind that nourishes both your body and your soul. But then, the familiar pang of gastroparesis hits, leaving you discouraged and unsure.

We know the struggle. Millions of women face the limitations of gastroparesis, and the joy of food can feel like a distant memory. But what if we told you it doesn't have to be this way?

This cookbook is your culinary rebellion. It's your declaration of independence from bland, uninspired meals. It's your passport to a world of vibrant flavors and textures, all designed specifically for women with gastroparesis.

Forget the frustration, the fear, and the endless internet searches for "safe" options. In these pages, you'll discover a revolution in your kitchen. We'll equip you with:

A symphony of taste: mouthwatering recipes for every meal, from quick and easy breakfasts to elegant dinners, all bursting with flavor and gentle on your digestion.

Beyond the recipe: Essential tips and tricks for meal planning, prepping, and navigating social situations – all while keeping your digestive health a top priority.

Empowerment through knowledge: We'll delve deeper into the science behind gastroparesis, answer your questions, and equip you to make informed choices about your diet.

This isn't just a cookbook; it's your guide to reclaiming your kitchen and rediscovering the pleasure of food. We'll transform mealtimes from struggles into celebrations of your strength and resilience.

Are you prepared to go on this gastronomic adventure? *Let's turn the limitations of gastroparesis into delicious possibilities.*

INTRODUCTION

Do you dream of delicious meals, but gastro paresis throws a wrench in your plans? Are you

tired of bland, boring food that leaves you uninspired? This cookbook is your invitation to a culinary revolution! Here, we rewrite the rules of gastro paresis cooking, transforming frustration into flavor.

Forget bland and boring! We'll show you how to create exciting dishes that tantalize your taste buds without upsetting your stomach. Whether you're newly diagnosed or a seasoned gastroparesis warrior, this book is your roadmap to a delicious and fulfilling life.

Inside, you'll find:

- ➢ **Gastro paresis Demystified:** We'll unveil the secrets of this condition, empowering you to understand your symptoms and take charge of your health.

- ➢ **Your Kitchen Transformed:** Discover essential pantry staples, navigate food labels with ease, and unlock clever cooking techniques to transform your kitchen into a gastro paresis-friendly haven.

- ➢ **A Culinary Adventure:** Embark on a flavor journey with a diverse collection of recipes. From energizing smoothies to comforting dinners, we'll show you how to create delicious meals for every occasion, all tailored for easy digestion.

- ➢ **Beyond the Kitchen:** We'll celebrate you! Explore tips for adapting recipes for holidays and gatherings, discover a supportive community of women who understand, and uncover resources to keep you motivated on your gastro paresis journey.

This book is your manual for rediscovering the love of cooking, not just a list of recipes. Let's turn mealtimes into celebrations, one delicious bite at a time. Are you ready to conquer your symptoms and savor flavor? ***Let's get started!***

Understanding Gastroparesis

Gastroparesis might sound intimidating, but with a little knowledge, you can take charge of your health and enjoy delicious meals again. Here's a breakdown of what it is, why it happens, and how it's diagnosed:

What is Gastroparesis?

Imagine your stomach as a muscular sac that squeezes and churns, breaking down food for your body to absorb nutrients. In gastroparesis, these muscles don't work as well as they should. This can lead to food sitting in your stomach for a longer time than usual, causing a variety of uncomfortable symptoms.

Causes of gastroparesis

Gastroparesis, a condition characterized by delayed stomach emptying, can significantly impact a patient's quality of life. While the exact cause often remains elusive, several factors can contribute to its development. ***Here's a breakdown of the prominent etiologies a medical professional should consider:***

Neutrogena Causes:

- ➢ **Diabetic Neuropathy:** This is the most common cause of gastro paresis. Chronic hyperglycemia in diabetes can damage the vague nerve, which controls stomach muscle contractions and emptying.
- ➢ **Idiopathic Gastroparesis:** In roughly 40% of cases, no clear cause can be identified. However, damage to the vague nerve from unknown origins is still suspected.
- ➢ **Post-Surgical Gastroparesis:** Surgery involving the stomach, esophagus, or vague nerve can lead to scar tissue formation or nerve damage, impacting stomach motility.

Other Medical Conditions:

- ➢ **Viral Infections:** Viral infections like cytomegalovirus (CMV) or norovirus can damage the nerves or muscles in the stomach, triggering gastro paresis.
- ➢ **Endocrine Disorders:** Hypothyroidism, a condition with low thyroid hormone levels, can contribute to delayed stomach emptying.
- ➢ **Autoimmune Disorders:** Scleroderma and amyloidosis, which affect connective tissues and protein deposits, respectively, can involve the stomach muscles or nerves, leading to gastro paresis.
- ➢ **Neurological Disorders:** Parkinson's disease and multiple sclerosis can affect the nervous system's control over the digestive tract, contributing to gastro paresis.

Miscellaneous Factors:

- ➢ **Gastrointestinal Motility Disorders:** Gastro esophageal reflux disease (GERD) and chronic intestinal pseudo-obstruction (CIPO) can sometimes present with symptoms like gastro paresis.
- ➢ **Certain Medications:** Opioid pain medications, tricyclic antidepressants, and anticholinergic drugs can have a side effect of slowing stomach emptying.
- ➢ It's crucial to conduct a thorough evaluation to identify the underlying cause of gastroparesis. This may involve a combination of tests like upper endoscopy, gastric emptying study, and blood tests to rule out other medical conditions.

Understanding the etiology of gastroparesis helps guide treatment decisions. For example, managing diabetes becomes crucial in diabetic gastroparesis, while addressing the underlying autoimmune disorder takes precedence in scleroderma-related cases.

Risk factors:

- ➢ **Nerve damage:** The vague nerve controls the muscles in your stomach. Damage to this nerve, often caused by diabetes, can disrupt the signals that tell your stomach to contract and move food along.
- ➢ **Viral infections:** In some cases, a viral infection can damage the nerves or muscles in your stomach, leading to gastroparesis.
- ➢ **Surgery:** Abdominal surgeries, especially those involving the vague nerve or stomach, can increase the risk of gastroparesis.
- ➢ **Certain medications:** Some medications, like narcotic pain relievers, can slow down stomach emptying.
- ➢ **Underlying conditions:** Gastroparesis can be associated with other conditions like hypothyroidism, amyloidosis (a buildup of protein in organs), and scleroderma (an autoimmune disease).

Symptoms and Diagnosis:

Gastroparesis can cause a range of symptoms, and their severity can vary from person to person.

Here are some common ones:

- **Nausea and vomiting:** Undigested food sitting in your stomach can trigger nausea and vomiting.

- **Feeling full after eating very little:** Since your stomach isn't emptying properly, you may feel a sense of fullness even after a small amount of food.

- **Abdominal pain and bloating:** Food trapped in your stomach can cause discomfort and bloating.

- **Weight loss:** Difficulty absorbing nutrients from food can lead to unintended weight loss.

- **Loss of appetite:** The feeling of fullness and nausea can make it hard to feel hungry.

Diagnosing Gastroparesis:

There's no **single test** for gastroparesis. Doctors typically use a combination of approaches, including:

- *Reviewing your medical history and symptoms:* Your doctor will ask about your symptoms, how long they've lasted, and any other medical conditions you may have.

- *Physical exam:* This may involve checking for signs of dehydration or malnutrition.

- *Imaging tests:* An X-ray or ultrasound can help rule out other problems like blockages in your digestive system.

- *Upper endoscopy:* A thin, flexible tube with a camera is inserted through your mouth to examine the inside of your stomach and esophagus.

- *Gastric emptying study:* This test involves eating a radioactive meal and using a special camera to track how quickly food leaves your stomach.

Managing Gastroparesis with Diet

Gastroparesis, a condition affecting stomach muscle function, can make mealtimes a challenge. However, a well-managed diet plays a crucial role in symptom control and overall well-being.

Here's a breakdown of why diet is important, what dietary guidelines to follow, and tips for meal planning with gastroparesis:

Importance of Diet In Gastroparesis Management:

A healthy diet becomes even more critical with gastroparesis. ***Here's why:***

Symptom Control: Certain foods slow down stomach emptying, worsening symptoms like nausea, vomiting, and bloating. A tailored diet can minimize these effects, improving your quality of life.

Nutrient Absorption: Delayed stomach emptying can hinder nutrient absorption. Consuming easily digestible foods ensures your body gets the essential vitamins and minerals it needs.

Maintaining Weight: Gastroparesis often leads to weight loss due to difficulty eating and nutrient malabsorption. A balanced diet helps maintain a healthy weight and supports overall health.

Dietary Guidelines for Gastroparesis:

Focus on Liquids and Soft Foods: Liquids and well-blended or puréed foods are easier for your stomach to digest and move through. Smoothies, soups, and mashed potatoes are good options.

Minimize Fiber: High-fiber foods can take longer to digest, causing discomfort. Choose low-fiber options like white bread, peeled fruits, and cooked vegetables.

Limit Fat: Dietary fat can slow down stomach emptying. opt for lean protein sources and low-fat cooking methods like baking, poaching, or grilling.

Smaller, More Frequent Meals: Eating smaller portions throughout the day reduces the burden on your stomach compared to a few large meals. Aim for 5-6 small meals or snacks spread evenly across the day.

Stay Hydrated: Gastroparesis can increase dehydration risk. Drink plenty of fluids throughout the day, choosing water over sugary drinks.

Tips for Meal Planning and Preparation:

Meal planning and preparation become essential tools for managing gastroparesis effectively.

Here are some tips:

Plan: Dedicate time each week to plan meals and create a grocery list based on your dietary needs.

Stock Up on Staples: Keep your pantry and fridge stocked with low-fiber and easily digestible options like canned fruits and vegetables, broth, protein shakes, and low-fat yogurt.

Prep in Advance: On good days, pre-cook or prep meals and snacks for later in the week. This guarantees you have wholesome options on hand and saves you time.

Pay Attention to Your Body: Observe how your body responds to various foods. Adjust your meal plan based on what triggers symptoms and what you tolerate well.

Consider Supplements: Talk to your doctor about vitamin or mineral supplements to address any nutritional deficiencies caused by gastroparesis.

By combining a tailored diet with other management strategies, you can effectively manage your gastroparesis and enjoy a healthy, fulfilling life.

MORNING MEALS

Soft and Easy-to-Digest Breakfast Options

Tropical Dream Smoothie

Ingredients:

- 1 frozen banana peeled and sliced.
- 1/2 cup low-fat yogurt (plain or vanilla)
- 1/4 cup low-fat milk
- 1/4 cup strained pineapple juice (or canned peaches/pears)
- 1/2 teaspoon ground cinnamon (optional)

Preparation Method:

- Combine all ingredients in a blender and process until smooth and creamy.
- Add a splash of low-fat milk or water if desired for a thinner consistency.

Total Preparation Time: 5 minutes

Nutrition Value
Calories: 200-250
Carbohydrates: 30-40 grams
Protein: 10-15 grams
Fat: 3-5 grams

Notes:

Substitute strained orange juice for pineapple juice if preferred but be mindful of acidity.

Feel free to add a sprinkle of ground ginger for a touch of spice.

Creamy Scrambled Eggs

Ingredients:

- 2 large eggs
- 1 tablespoon low-fat milk or water
- 1/2 teaspoon butter or olive oil
- Salt and pepper to taste

Preparation Method:

- In a bowl, whisk together eggs and milk or water. Season with salt and pepper.
- In a nonstick pan, heat up some oil or butter over medium flame.
- Pour in the egg mixture and cook, gently stirring with a spatula, until the eggs are set to your desired consistency.
- Serve immediately.

Cooking Time: 3-5 minutes

Total Preparation Time: 5 minutes

Nutrition Value
Calories: 140-160
Carbohydrates: 1-2 grams
Protein: 12-14 grams
Fat: 7-9 grams

<u>Notes:</u>

For a creamier texture, add a dollop of low-fat ricotta cheese or cottage cheese after cooking. Chopped cooked vegetables like spinach or chopped cooked mushrooms can be added for extra flavor and nutrients.

<u>Mashed Potato Power Bowl</u>

Ingredients:

- 1 medium potato peeled and diced.
- 1/4 cup low-fat milk or broth
- 1/4 cup cooked, shredded lean protein (chicken, fish, or turkey)
- 1/4 cup well-cooked, chopped vegetables (carrots, green beans, zucchini)
- Salt and pepper to taste

Preparation Method:

- In a pot, boil the diced potato until tender. Remove the seeds and mash them smooth using milk or broth. Season with salt and pepper.
- In a separate pan, heat a touch of oil and cook the chosen protein until heated through.
- In a bowl, combine mashed potatoes, cooked protein, chopped vegetables, and additional

salt and pepper to taste.

Cooking Time: 10-15 minutes (potato boiling) + Protein cooking time.

Total Preparation Time: 15-20 minutes

Nutrition Value:
Calories: 300-350
Carbohydrates: 30-40 grams
Protein: 20-25 grams
Fat: 5-7 grams

Notes:

This recipe is a base, feel free to add other gastroparesis-friendly toppings like crumbled low-fiber crackers or a dollop of low-fat yogurt.

Leftover cooked vegetables from another recipe can be used to save time.

Apple & Cinnamon Delight

Ingredients:

- One medium apple, cored, chopped, and weighed out at roughly one cup.
- 1/2 cup water
- 1/4 cup unsweetened applesauce
- 1/2 teaspoon ground cinnamon
- 1/4 teaspoon lemon juice (optional)
- Pinch of ground nutmeg (optional)

Preparation Method:

- In a saucepan, combine the diced apple, water, applesauce, and cinnamon.
- Bring to a simmer over medium heat. Cook for 5-7 minutes, or until the apples are tender.
- Take off the heat and add the lemon juice, if using.
- Using an immersion blender or food processor, partially puree the mixture until it reaches a desired consistency (smooth or slightly chunky). Alternatively, you can mash the apples with a fork for a more rustic texture.

Cooking Time: 5-7 minutes

Total Preparation Time: 10 minutes

Portion Size: 1 serving.

Nutrition Value (approximate per serving):
Calories: 70
Carbohydrates: 17g
Fiber: 2g
Sugar: 14g (natural sugar from apples and applesauce)
Fat: 0g
Protein: 0.5g

Notes:

You can adjust the amount of water depending on your desired consistency.

Feel free to add a pinch of ground nutmeg for additional flavor.

This recipe can be served warm or chilled.

Simple White Toast with Avocado

Ingredients:

- 1 slice white bread, toasted.
- 1/2 ripe avocado, mashed.
- Squeeze of lemon juice (optional)
- Pinch of salt and pepper (to taste)

Preparation Method:

- Toast a slice of white bread to your desired level of doneness.
- Mash the ripe avocado with a fork until smooth.
- Spread the mashed avocado on the toast.
- Add a squeeze of lemon juice (if using) for a brighter flavor.
- Add a dash of pepper and salt to taste.

Cooking Time: Toasting time will vary depending on your toaster.

Total Preparation Time: 5 minutes

Portion Size: 1 serving.

Nutrition Value (approximate per serving):

Calories: 180
Carbohydrates: 22g
Fiber: 3g
Sugar: 1g
Fat: 10g (healthy fats from avocado)
Protein: 2g

Notes:

You can use any type of white bread you prefer.

For a richer flavor, drizzle a touch of olive oil on the toast before adding the avocado.

Nutrient-Dense Smoothies and Shakes:

Green Power Smoothie:

Ingredients:

- 1 medium banana (ripe or frozen)
- 2 cups spinach (fresh or frozen)
- 1 cup chopped, peeled cantaloupe or honeydew melon.
- 1 cup low-fat milk or unsweetened plant-based milk (e.g., almond milk)
- Optional: 1 scoop vanilla protein powder (check for low-fiber content)

Preparation Method:

- Combine all ingredients in a blender and process until smooth and creamy.

Total Preparation Time: 5 minutes

Portion Size: 1 serving (approximately 2 cups)

Nutrition Value:
Calories: 250-350 (depending on protein powder)
Protein: 10-20g (with protein powder)
Carbohydrates: 40-50g
Fat: 5-10g (depending on milk choice)
Fiber: Less than 2g

Tropical Paradise Shake:

Ingredients:

- 1 cup chopped, peeled ripe banana.

- 1 cup chopped, peeled mango (fresh or frozen)

- 1/2 cup strained pineapple juice (unsweetened)

- 1 cup low-fat yogurt or unsweetened plant-based yogurt (e.g., coconut yogurt)

- 1/2 cup low-fat milk or unsweetened plant-based milk (e.g., coconut milk)

Preparation Method:

- Combine all ingredients in a blender and process until smooth and creamy.

Total Preparation Time: 5 minutes

Portion Size: 1 serving (approximately 2 cups)

Nutrition Value:
Calories: 250-300
Protein: 8-10g (with yogurt)
Carbohydrates: 45-50g
Fat: 5-10g (depending on milk and yogurt choice)
Fiber: Less than 2g

Banana Berry Boost:

Ingredients:

- 1 cup chopped, peeled ripe banana (fresh or frozen)
- 1/2 cup strained mixed berries (e.g., blueberries, raspberries) - optional (check for low-fiber options)
- 1 cup low-fat yogurt or unsweetened plant-based yogurt (e.g., soy yogurt)
- 1 cup low-fat milk or unsweetened plant-based milk (e.g., oat milk)
- Optional: 1/4 cup low-sugar applesauce (for additional sweetness)

Preparation Method:

- If using berries, strain them to minimize pulp.
- Combine all ingredients in a blender and process until smooth and creamy.

Total Preparation Time: 5 minutes

Portion Size: 1 serving (approximately 2 cups)

Nutrition Value:
Calories: 200-250
Protein: 8-10g (with yogurt)
Carbohydrates: 40-50g (depending on berries and applesauce)
Fat: 5-10g (depending on milk and yogurt choice)
Fiber: Less than 2g (without berries)

Creamy Vanilla Delight

Ingredients:

- 1 cup low-fat yogurt (plain or vanilla)
- 1/2 banana, frozen and sliced.
- 1/2 cup low-fat milk
- 1 teaspoon honey (optional)
- 1/4 teaspoon vanilla extract

Preparation Method:

- In a blender, combine the frozen banana slices, low-fat yogurt, milk, honey (if using), and vanilla extract.

- Blend until smooth and creamy.
- Pour into a glass and enjoy.

Total Preparation Time: 5 minutes

Portion Size: 1 serving.

Nutrition Value (approximate per serving):
Calories: 180-200 (depending on the yogurt and use of honey)
Protein: 10-12 grams
Carbohydrates: 25-30 grams
Fat: 3-5 grams

Cantaloupe Cooler

Ingredients:

- 2 cups diced cantaloupe.
- 1/2 cup water
- 1/4 cup low-fat milk (optional)
- Few sprigs of mint (optional)
- Lime wedge (optional)

Preparation Method:

- In a blender, combine the diced cantaloupe and water.
- Blend until smooth.
- If preferred, strain the mixture to get rid of any pulp.
- Add low-fat milk for a creamier consistency (optional).
- Pour into a glass and garnish with a mint sprig and/or lime wedge (optional).

Total Preparation Time: 5 minutes

Portion Size: 1 serving.

Nutrition Value (approximate per serving):
Calories: 40-50
Protein: 1 gram

Carbohydrates: 10-12 grams
Fat: trace amount
Porridges and hot cereals:

Creamy Rice Delight

Ingredients:

- 1 cup cooked white rice.
- 1 cup low-fat cream soup (or 1/2 cup low-fat yogurt and 1/4 cup shredded low-fat cheese)
- 1/2 cup low-fat milk or broth
- 1/4 cup chopped cooked carrots (optional)
- Salt and pepper to taste (optional)
- Fresh herbs like chopped parsley or chives for garnish (optional)

Preparation Method:

- In a saucepan, heat the low-fat milk or broth over medium heat.
- Stir in the cooked white rice and cream soup (or yogurt and cheese mixture).
- If using, add the chopped cooked carrots.
- Heat through, stirring occasionally, until warmed and creamy. (Approximately 5 minutes)
- If preferred, add salt and pepper to taste.
- Garnish with fresh herbs (optional) before serving.

Cooking Time: 5 minutes

Total Preparation Time: 10 minutes (including cooking rice)

Portion Size: 1 serving.

Nutrition Value (approximate per serving):
Calories: 300-400 (depending on cream soup/yogurt choice)
Carbohydrates: 40-50g
Protein: 10-15g
Fat: 5-10g

Simple White Rice with Scrambled Egg

Ingredients:

- 1/2 cup cooked white rice.

- 1 egg

- 1 tablespoon low-fat milk or water

- Pinch of salt and pepper to taste

- Non-stick cooking spray

Preparation Method:

- In a bowl, whisk together the egg, milk or water, and salt and pepper.

- Apply cooking spray to a nonstick pan and heat it over medium heat.

- Pour in the egg mixture and scramble until cooked through, stirring frequently.

- In a separate bowl, combine the cooked white rice and scrambled eggs.

- Gently mix to combine and warm through for a minute.

Cooking Time: 5 minutes (including cooking rice)

Total Preparation Time: 10 minutes

Portion Size: 1 serving.

Nutrition Value (approximate per serving):
Calories: 200-250
Carbohydrates: 30-40g
Protein: 10-12g
Fat: 5-7g

Mashed Potato & Veggie Mash up.

Ingredients:

- 1 medium potato peeled and cubed.

- 1/2 cup well-cooked vegetables (options: carrots, green beans, zucchini)

- 1/4 cup low-fat milk or broth

- Salt and pepper to taste

- A pat of butter or a light coating of olive oil (optional)

Preparation Method:

- In a pot, cover the cubed potato with water and bring to a boil.

- Reduce heat and simmer until the potato is tender (approximately 15-20 minutes).

- While the potato cooks, steam or boil the chosen vegetables until tender.

- Drain the water from the potato and mash it with a fork or potato masher.

- On top of the mashed potato, add the cooked veggies.

- Mash together until well combined.

- Stir in the low-fat milk or broth until desired consistency is reached.

- Season with salt and pepper to taste.

- For extra flavor, add a pat of butter or drizzle of olive oil (optional).

Cooking Time: 20–25 minutes

Total Preparation Time: 30 minutes

Portion Size: 1 serving.

Nutrition Value (approximate per serving):
Calories: 150-200 (depending on added butter/oil)
Carbohydrates: 30-40g
Protein: 2-3g
Fat: 5-10g (depending on added butter/oil)

Tropical Dream Smoothie

Ingredients:

- 1 cup peeled and seeded ripe banana, frozen.
- ½ cup strained mango juice
- ½ cup strained pineapple juice (avoid if acidic)
- ¼ cup cooked white rice
- ½ cup low-fat yogurt (plain or with low-fiber fruit puree)

Preparation Method:

- Combine all ingredients in a blender and process until smooth and creamy.
- Add a splash of low-fat milk or water if needed for desired consistency.

Total Preparation Time: 5 minutes

Portion Size: 1 serving.

Nutrition Value:
Calories: 250
Carbohydrates: 45g
Protein: 5g
Fat: 2g

Berry Blast Breakfast Bowl

Ingredients:

- ½ cup cooked white rice
- ½ cup low-fat yogurt (plain or with low-fiber fruit puree)
- ¼ cup puffed rice cereal
- ¼ cup sliced ripe strawberries
- ¼ cup blueberries

Preparation Method:

- In a bowl, combine cooked white rice and low-fat yogurt.
- Top with puffed rice cereal, sliced strawberries, and blueberries.

Total Preparation Time: 5 minutes

Portion Size: 1 serving.

Nutrition Value:
Calories: 200
Carbohydrates: 40g
Protein: 5g
Fat: 2g

Low-Fiber Breads and Toast Toppings:

<u>Mashed Avocado Toast</u>

Ingredients:

- 1 slice white bread (toasted)
- 1/2 ripe avocado
- Squeeze of lemon juice (optional)
- Pinch of salt (optional)
- Pinch of red pepper flakes (optional)

Preparation Method:

- Toast the white bread slice to your desired level of crispness.
- Using a fork, mash the avocado until the appropriate consistency is achieved.
- Spread the mashed avocado on the toasted bread.
- Add a squeeze of lemon juice, salt, and red pepper flakes (optional) for additional flavor.

Total Preparation Time: 5 minutes

Portion Size: 1 slice of toast.

Nutrition Value (approximate):
Calories: 220
Fat: 14g
Carbohydrates: 22g
Protein: 3g
Fiber: 4g (depending on avocado ripeness)

Cream Cheese Delight

Ingredients:

- 1/2 cup low-fat yogurt (plain or flavored)
- 1 tablespoon low-fat cream cheese, softened.
- 1/4 cup chopped, low-fiber fruit (e.g., cantaloupe, honeydew melon, skinned canned peaches/pears)
- Optional toppings: Chopped nuts (limited amounts), ground cinnamon

Preparation Method:

- In a bowl, combine the low-fat yogurt and cream cheese. Mix well until smooth and creamy.
- Fold in the chopped fruit.
- Top with chopped nuts (optional) and sprinkle with ground cinnamon (optional) for added flavor.

Total Preparation Time: 5 minutes

Portion Size: 1 serving.

Nutrition Value (approximate):
Calories: 130
Fat: 3g
Carbohydrates: 18g
Protein: 5g
Fiber: 1g (depending on fruit)

Yogurt Berry Surprise

Ingredients:

- 1/2 cup low-fat yogurt (plain or flavored)
- 1/4 cup strained fruit juice (e.g., peach, pear)
- 1 tablespoon mashed banana

Preparation Method:

- In a bowl, combine the low-fat yogurt and strained fruit juice. Mix well.

- Gently fold in the mashed banana to create a marbled effect.

Total Preparation Time: 5 minutes

Portion Size: 1 serving.

Nutrition Value (approximate):
Calories: 110
Fat: 0g
Carbohydrates: 22g
Protein: 5g
Fiber: 1g (depending on banana ripeness)

<u>Yogurt and Nut Butter Parfait</u>

Ingredients:

- 1/2 cup low-fat yogurt (plain or flavored)

- 2 tablespoons nut butter (peanut butter, almond butter, etc.)

- 1/4 cup sliced banana.

- 1 tablespoon honey

- Optional: Chopped nuts for garnish

Preparation Method:

- In a small bowl or parfait glass, layer half of the yogurt.

- Top with half of the sliced banana.

- Drizzle with 1 teaspoon of honey.

- Add a tablespoon of nut butter.

- Repeat layers with remaining yogurt, banana, honey, and nut butter.

- (Optional) Top with chopped nuts for garnish.

Total Preparation Time: 5 minutes

Portion Size: 1 serving.

Nutrition Information (approximate):

Nutrition Information
Calories: 250-350 (depending on the type of yogurt and nut butter used)
Fat: 10-15g
Carbohydrates: 30-40g
Protein: 10-15g

Sliced Apple with Nut Butter and Honey Drizzle

Ingredients:

- 1 apple cored and sliced.
- 2 tablespoons nut butter (peanut butter, almond butter, etc.)
- 1 tablespoon honey

Preparation Method:

- Slice the apple into thin wedges or bite-sized pieces.
- Spread nut butter on each apple slice.
- Drizzle honey over the apple slices.

Total Preparation Time: 2 minutes

Portion Size: 1 serving.

Nutrition Information (approximate):
Calories: 150-200 (depending on the size of the apple)
Fat: 5-10g
Carbohydrates: 20-30g
Protein: 2-3g

Light and Nourishing Soups

Creamy Carrot Soup

Ingredients:

- 2 tablespoons olive oil
- 1 medium onion, chopped.
- 2 pounds carrots peeled and sliced.
- 4 cups low-sodium chicken broth
- 1 cup water
- 1/2 teaspoon ground ginger
- 1/4 teaspoon ground nutmeg
- Salt and pepper to taste
- 1/2 cup low-fat yogurt (optional)

Preparation Method:

- In a big pot, warm up the olive oil over medium heat. Add onions and cook until softened, about 5 minutes.
- Add carrots, chicken broth, water, ginger, and nutmeg. Once the carrots are soft, bring to a boil, lower the heat, and simmer for 20 to 25 minutes.
- Allow the soup to cool a little. Smoothly mix the soup in batches in a blender. Additionally, you can use an immersion blender within the cooker.
- After adding the soup back to the pot, adjust the seasoning with salt and pepper.
- If using yogurt for a creamier texture, stir in the yogurt and heat gently until warmed through. (Optional)

Cooking Time: 30 minutes

Total Preparation Time: 35 minutes (including chopping vegetables)

Portion Size: 1 cup.

Nutrition Value (per serving):

Calories: 150, Fat: 5g, Carbohydrates: 20g, Protein: 5g, Sodium (depending on broth): 400mg

Chicken Noodle Soup

Ingredients:

- 2 tablespoons olive oil
- 1 medium onion, chopped.
- 1 carrot peeled and diced.
- 1 celery stalk, diced.
- 4 cups low-sodium chicken broth
- 4 cups water
- 1pound boneless, skinless chicken breasts, chopped.
- 1/2 cup low-fiber pasta (like white rice or corn noodles)
- 1 teaspoon dried thyme
- 1/2 teaspoon dried parsley
- Salt and pepper to taste

Preparation Method:

- In a large pot set over medium heat, warm the olive oil. Add onions, carrots, and celery. Cook until softened, about 5 minutes.
- Add chicken broth, water, chicken breasts, thyme, and parsley. When the chicken is cooked through, simmer it for 15 to 20 minutes over low heat after bringing it to a boil.
- Add pasta and simmer for an additional 5-7 minutes, or until pasta is cooked according to package directions.
- Season with salt and pepper to taste.

Cooking Time: 30 minutes

Total Preparation Time: 35 minutes (including chopping vegetables)

Portion Size: 1 cup.

Nutrition Value (per serving):

Calories: 250, Fat: 5g, Carbohydrates: 30g, Protein: 20g, Sodium (depending on broth): 400mg

Tomato Bisque (without Cream)

Ingredients:

- 2 tablespoons olive oil
- 1 medium onion, chopped.
- 2 cloves garlic, minced.
- 1 (28-ounce) can crushed tomatoes (preferably low-sodium)
- 4 cups low-sodium chicken broth
- 1/2 cup of freshly chopped basil (or 1 teaspoon of dried basil)
- 1/4 teaspoon dried oregano
- Salt and pepper to taste
- 1 tablespoon cornstarch (optional)

Preparation Method:

- In a big pot set over medium heat, warm the olive oil. Cook the garlic and onions for five minutes or until they are tender.
- Incorporate the smashed tomatoes, oregano, basil, and chicken broth. After bringing to a boil, lower heat, and simmer for 20 minutes.
- Puree the soup until smooth, either in batches in a standard blender or with an immersion blender.
- After adding the soup back to the pot, adjust the seasoning with salt and pepper. If you prefer a thicker soup, mix the cornstarch with a tablespoon of water to create a slurry. Stir the slurry into the soup and simmer for a few minutes until thickened. (Optional)

Cooking Time: 30 minutes

Total Preparation Time: 35 minutes (including chopping vegetables)

Portion Size: 1 cup.

Nutrition Value (per serving):
Calories: 120, Fat: 3g, Carbohydrates: 20g, Protein: 5g, Sodium (depending on broth): 40

Creamy Potato Soup

Ingredients:

- 3 tablespoons unsalted butter
- One diced medium yellow onion (about 1.5 cups)
- Three large cloves of minced garlic and four cups of low-sodium vegetable or chicken

broth

- Two pounds of chopped and peeled russet potatoes (approximately six cups)
- 1 teaspoon dried thyme
- 1/2 teaspoon salt
- 1/4 teaspoon black pepper
- 1 1/2 cups low-fat milk
- 1/2 cup shredded cheddar cheese (optional)
- Chopped fresh chives, for garnish (optional)

Preparation Method:

- Melt butter over medium heat in a big pot or Dutch oven. When the onion is tender, add it and simmer for about five minutes. Add the minced garlic and simmer, stirring, for one more minute, until aromatic.
- Add the chicken broth, diced potatoes, thyme, salt, and pepper. Bring to a boil, then reduce heat and simmer for 15-20 minutes, or until the potatoes are tender.

- Puree the soup until smooth, either with an immersion blender or in batches using a blender. You can also leave the soup partially chunky, depending on your preference.
- Stir in the low-fat milk and heat through, about 2-3 minutes. Remove from heat and stir in shredded cheddar cheese, if using.
- If preferred, add more salt and pepper to taste and adjust the seasonings.

Cooking Time: 20-25 minutes

Total Preparation Time: 30 minutes

Portion Size: 1 cup.

Nutrition Value per Serving (approximate):
Calories: 250
Fat: 10g
Saturated Fat: 6g
Cholesterol: 30mg
Sodium: 450mg (depending on broth used)

| Carbohydrates: 30g |
| Fiber: 2g |
| Sugar: 5g |
| Protein: 10g |

Notes:

You can substitute vegetable broth for chicken broth for a vegan option.

For a richer flavor, you can use heavy cream instead of low-fat milk, but this will increase the calorie and fat content.

Feel free to add other vegetables to the soup, such as chopped carrots, celery, or green beans.

Vegetable Garden Soup

Ingredients:

- 1 tablespoon olive oil
- 1 medium onion, chopped (about 1.5 cups)
- 2 carrots peeled and diced.
- 2 celery stalks, diced.
- 2 cloves garlic, minced.
- 4 cups low-sodium vegetable broth
- 1 (14.5 oz) can diced tomatoes, undrained
- 1 cup frozen peas
- 1 cup chopped green beans.
- 1 cup chopped zucchini.
- 1/2 teaspoon dried oregano
- 1/4 teaspoon dried basil
- Salt and black pepper to taste
- Chopped fresh parsley, for garnish (optional)

Preparation Method:

- Olive oil should be heated over medium heat in a big pot or Dutch oven. Add the chopped onion, carrots, and celery. Cook until softened, about 5-7 minutes. Add the minced garlic and simmer for one more minute after stirring.

- Add the vegetable broth, diced tomatoes (with their juices), frozen peas, green beans, zucchini, oregano, and basil. Bring to a boil, then reduce heat and simmer for 15-20 minutes, or until the vegetables are tender-crisp.

- Add a dash of black pepper and salt to taste.

Cooking Time: 20-25 minutes

Total Preparation Time: 30 minutes

Portion Size: 1 cup.

Nutrition Value per serving (approximate):
Calories: 150
Fat: 5g
Saturated Fat: 1g
Cholesterol: 0mg
Sodium: 400mg (depending on broth used)
Carbohydrates: 25g
Fiber: 5g
Sugar: 5g
Protein: 5g

<u>Notes:</u>

You can add other vegetables to the soup, such as chopped mushrooms, corn, or bell peppers.

To make the soup thicker, you can mash some of the cooked vegetables with a fork before adding them back to the pot.

If you prefer a smoother soup, you can use an immersion blender to puree some of the vegetables.

Protein-Rich Sandwiches and Wraps:

<u>Turkey & Avocado Wrap</u>

Ingredients:

- Two large, cleaned, and dried romaine lettuce leaves
- 3 ounces sliced, cooked, lean ground turkey or shredded cooked chicken breast.
- 1/4 ripe avocado, mashed.
- 1 tablespoon low-fat mayonnaise (optional)
- 1 tablespoon chopped red onion (optional)
- Salt and pepper to taste

Preparation Method:

- Spread mashed avocado on one romaine lettuce leaf.
- Top with sliced turkey or chicken, red onion (if using), and a sprinkle of salt and pepper.
- Drizzle with low-fat mayonnaise (if using) for added creaminess.
- Roll up the lettuce leaf with the filling inside.

Total Preparation Time: 5 minutes

Nutrition Value (estimated):
Calories: 250-300 (depending on the use of mayonnaise)
Protein: 20-25 grams
Fat: 10-15 grams (higher with mayonnaise)
Carbohydrates: 5-10 grams
Fiber: 2-3 grams

Egg Salad Sandwich

Ingredients:

- 2 slices white bread, toasted (optional)
- 2 hard-boiled eggs, chopped.
- 1 tablespoon low-fat mayonnaise
- 1 tablespoon chopped celery (optional)
- 1/4 teaspoon dried dill (optional)
- Salt and pepper to taste

Preparation Method:

- In a bowl, combine chopped eggs, mayonnaise, celery (if using), dill (if using), salt, and pepper.
- Spread the egg salad mixture on one slice of toasted bread (if using).
- Top with the other slice of bread.

Cooking Time: Boiling eggs - 10-12 minutes (depending on desired doneness)

Total Preparation Time: 15 minutes (including boiling eggs)

Nutrition Value (estimated):
Calories: 250-300 (depending on the use of toast)
Protein: 15-20 grams
Fat: 10-15 grams
Carbohydrates: 20-25 grams (higher with toast)
Fiber: 2-3 grams (higher with celery)

Creamy Chicken Salad

Ingredients:

- 3 ounces cooked, shredded chicken breast.
- 1/4 ripe avocado, mashed.
- 1 tablespoon low-fat Greek yogurt
- 1 tablespoon chopped red onion (optional)
- 1/4 teaspoon dried parsley (optional)
- Salt and pepper to taste

Preparation Method:

- In a bowl, combine shredded chicken, mashed avocado, Greek yogurt, red onion (if using), parsley (if using), salt, and pepper.
- Mix well until creamy and combined.

Cooking Time: Cooking chicken - varies depending on method (baking, poaching, etc.)

Total Preparation Time: 10 minutes (assuming pre-cooked chicken)

Nutrition Value (estimated):
Calories: 250-300

Protein: 25-30 grams
Fat: 10-15 grams
Carbohydrates: 5-10 grams
Fiber: 2-3 grams

<u>Tofu Scramble Wrap</u>

Ingredients:

- 14 oz block firm tofu, pressed for at least 30 minutes.
- 1 tablespoon nutritional yeast
- 1 teaspoon turmeric powder
- ½ teaspoon garlic powder
- 1 tablespoon olive oil
- ½ medium onion, chopped
- 4 oz mushrooms, sliced (optional)
- ½ cup chopped spinach or kale (or a mix)
- 2 whole wheat tortillas
- Salt and pepper to taste
- Optional toppings: Sliced avocado, salsa, vegan cheese

Preparation Method:

- ➢ *Cook the Tofu Scramble:* Crumble the pressed tofu using your fingers or a fork. In a bowl, toss the crumbled tofu with nutritional yeast, turmeric powder, and garlic powder.
- ➢ *Cook the Veggies:* In a big skillet set over medium heat, add the olive oil. Cook for about five minutes, or until the chopped onion is tender. If using, add the sliced mushrooms and cook for an additional 2-3 minutes.
- ➢ *Add the Tofu:* Add the crumbled tofu mixture to the pan with the vegetables. Stir-fry for 5-7 minutes, breaking up any large tofu chunks, until golden brown and heated through.
- ➢ *Season and Add Greens:* Season the tofu scramble with salt and pepper to taste. Add the chopped spinach or kale and cook for another minute, until wilted.
- ➢ *Assemble the Wrap:* Warm the tortillas in a dry skillet or microwave for a few seconds. Spread the tofu scramble mixture evenly over each tortilla. Add your desired toppings

like sliced avocado, salsa, or vegan cheese.

> ➤ *Fold and Serve:* Fold the tortillas in half or roll them up burrito-style. Serve immediately.

Cooking Time: 10-15 minutes

Total Preparation Time: 15-20 minutes

Portion Size: 1 wrap.

Nutrition Value (approximate per serving):
Calories: 350-400
Protein: 20-25 grams
Carbohydrates: 30-35 grams
Fat: 15-20 grams

Notes:

Depending on your taste, you can change the quantity of spices.

Feel free to add other vegetables to the tofu scramble, such as chopped bell peppers, zucchini, or tomatoes.

Use a non-stick pan for easier cleaning.

Tuna Salad Pita

Ingredients:

- 5 oz canned tuna in water, drained.
- 2 tablespoons low-fat mayonnaise
- 1 stalk celery finely chopped.
- ¼ red onion, finely chopped
- 1 tablespoon chopped fresh dill (optional)
- Salt and pepper to taste
- 1 whole wheat pita bread
- Optional toppings: Lettuce or spinach leaves, sliced tomato, cucumber slices

Preparation Method:

- Make the Tuna Salad: In a bowl, combine the drained tuna, mayonnaise, chopped celery, red onion, and dill (if using). Season with salt and pepper to taste.
- Prepare the Pita: Warm the whole wheat pita bread in a dry skillet or microwave for a

few seconds to soften. You can also cut the pita bread in half to create a pocket.

- Assemble the Pita: Fill the warmed pita bread with the tuna salad mixture. Add your desired toppings like lettuce or spinach leaves, sliced tomato, and cucumber slices.

Cooking Time: 2-3 minutes

Total Preparation Time: 5-10 minutes

Portion Size: 1 pita.

Nutrition Value (approximate per serving):
Calories: 300-350
Protein: 25-30 grams
Carbohydrates: 30-35 grams
Fat: 10-15 grams

Notes:

You can use canned tuna in olive oil instead of water but adjust the total fat content accordingly.

Feel free to add other chopped vegetables to the tuna salad, such as carrots, bell peppers, or green beans.

If you don't have fresh dill, you can use a pinch of dried dill weed.

Satisfying Side Dishes and Accompaniments:

Mashed Potatoes with Herbs

Ingredients:

- 2 medium russet potatoes peeled and cubed.
- 1 cup low-fat milk (or low-sodium broth)
- 1/4 cup chopped fresh herbs (parsley, chives, thyme, or a combination)
- 1 tablespoon unsalted butter
- Salt and black pepper to taste

Preparation:

- In a medium pot, cover potatoes with water and bring to a boil. After lowering the heat, simmer the potatoes for 15 to 20 minutes, or until a fork pierce them easily. Thoroughly drain potatoes.

- Mashing: Put potatoes back in the pot and use a potato masher to mash them until they are largely smooth. Gradually add low-fat milk (or broth) while mashing until desired consistency is reached.
- Flavoring: Stir in chopped herbs, butter, salt, and pepper to taste. Serve immediately.

Total Preparation Time: 25 minutes

Cooking Time: 15-20 minutes

Nutrition Value (per serving):
Calories: Approximately 200 kcal
Carbohydrates: Approximately 35 g
Protein: Approximately 5 g
Fat: Approximately 5 g (depending on butter amount)

Roasted White Rice

Ingredients:

- 1 cup white rice, rinsed.
- 1 ½ cups low-sodium chicken broth (or vegetable broth)
- 1 tablespoon olive oil
- Salt and pepper to taste

Preparation:

- Preheat oven to 375°F (190°C). In a baking dish, combine rinsed rice, broth, olive oil, salt, and pepper.
- Baking: Cover the dish with foil and bake for 20 minutes or until rice is cooked through and all liquid is absorbed. Fluff with a fork before serving.

Total Preparation Time: 30 minutes

Cooking Time: 20 minutes

Nutrition Value (per serving):
Calories: Approximately 200 kcal
Carbohydrates: Approximately 40 g

Protein: Approximately 3 g

Fat: Approximately 3 g (depending on olive oil amount)

Sautéed Green Beans with Garlic

Ingredients:

- 1 cup fresh green beans, trimmed and cut into bite-sized pieces.
- 1 tablespoon olive oil
- 1 clove garlic, minced.
- Salt and pepper to taste

Preparation:

- Heat olive oil in a pan over medium heat. Add garlic and cook for 30 seconds, until fragrant.
- Sautéing: Add green beans to the pan and cook for 5-7 minutes, or until tender-crisp, stirring occasionally. Season with salt and pepper to taste.

Total Preparation Time: 10 minutes

Cooking Time: 5-7 minutes

Nutrition Value (per serving):
Calories: Approximately 50 kcal
Carbohydrates: Approximately 8 g
Protein: Approximately 1 g
Fat: Approximately 3 g (depending on olive oil amount)

Steamed Zucchini with Lemon

Ingredients:

- 2 medium zucchini (around 10 oz total)
- 1 tablespoon olive oil
- 1/2 teaspoon salt

- 1/4 teaspoon freshly ground black pepper.

- 1 lemon, juiced (about 2 tablespoons)

- 1 tablespoon fresh parsley, chopped (optional)

Preparation Method:

- Wash and trim the ends of the zucchini. Slice them into rounds or half-moons, about 1/4-inch thick.

- In a large pot, bring about 1 inch of water to a boil.

- While the water is heating, in a small bowl, whisk together the olive oil, salt, and pepper.

- Add a steamer basket to the pot, ensuring it doesn't touch the boiling water. Alternatively, use a colander placed over the pot.

- Place the zucchini slices in the steamer basket.

- Cover the pot and steam the zucchini for 3-5 minutes, or until tender-crisp. The exact time may vary depending on the thickness of your slices.

- Once cooked, transfer the zucchini to a serving dish.

- Drizzle with the prepared lemon juice and olive oil mixture.

- Garnish with chopped parsley (optional) and serve immediately.

Cooking Time: 3-5 minutes

Total Preparation Time: 10 minutes

Portion Size: 1 serving (around 5 oz zucchini)

Nutrition Value (per serving):
Calories: 40 kcal
Fat: 3 g
Saturated Fat: 0.5 g
Cholesterol: 0 mg
Sodium: 140 mg (depending on salt added)
Carbohydrates: 5 g
Fiber: 1 g
Sugar: 2 g

Protein: 1 g

<u>Applesauce</u>

Ingredients:

- 3-4 medium apples (around 1.5 lbs. total)

- 1/4 cup water

- 1 tablespoon lemon juice (optional)

- 1/4 teaspoon ground cinnamon (optional)

Preparation Method:

- Wash, core, and cut the apples into chunks.

- In a medium saucepan, combine the apples, water, and lemon juice (if using).

- Put the mixture on medium heat and bring it to a boil.

- Reduce heat to low, cover the pan, and simmer for 15-20 minutes, or until the apples are softened.

- Take the pan off from the burner and allow the apples to cool slightly.

- Using an immersion blender or a food processor, puree the applesauce to your desired consistency. You can leave it slightly chunky or puree it completely smooth.

- Stir in the ground cinnamon (if using) and taste. Adjust sweetness with additional lemon juice or a touch of honey if desired.

- Let the applesauce cool completely before serving. Leftover applesauce keeps for up to five days in the refrigerator when kept in an airtight container.

Cooking Time: 15-20 minutes

Total Preparation Time: 25 minutes

Portion Size: 1/2 cup (around 4 oz)

Nutrition Value (per 1/2 cup serving):
Calories: 60 kcal
Fat: 0.5 g
Saturated Fat: 0 g
Cholesterol: 0 mg
Sodium: 2 mg
Carbohydrates: 15 g
Fiber: 2 g
Sugar: 12 g (naturally occurring sugars)
Protein: 0.5 g

DELICIOUS DINNERS

Tender and Flavorful Meat and Poultry Dishes

Creamy Chicken and Rice

Ingredients:

- 1 tablespoon olive oil
- One pound of bite-sized, deboned, and skinless chicken breasts
- 1/2 onion, chopped.
- 1 clove garlic, minced.
- 1 teaspoon dried thyme
- 1/4 teaspoon salt
- 1/4 teaspoon black pepper
- 2 cups low-sodium chicken broth
- 1 cup cooked white rice.
- 1 (10.5-ounce) can condensed cream of chicken soup (low-fat or fat-free)
- 1/4 cup chopped cooked carrots (optional)
- Chopped fresh parsley (for garnish, optional)

Preparation Method:

- Place olive oil in a big skillet and heat it over medium heat. Add chicken and cook until golden brown on all sides, about 5-7 minutes.
- Stir in onion, garlic, thyme, salt, and pepper. Cook for 1 minute more, until softened.
- Add chicken broth and bring to a simmer. Remove any browned residue from the pan's bottom by scraping it up.
- Stir in cooked white rice and cream of chicken soup. After lowering the heat to low, simmer the chicken for ten minutes, or until it is thoroughly cooked.
- If using, stir in chopped cooked carrots during the last minute of simmering.
- Serve garnished with chopped fresh parsley (optional).

Cooking Time: 20 minutes

Total Preparation Time: 25 minutes

Nutrition Value per serving (approximate):
Calories: 400
Fat: 12g
Carbohydrates: 45g
Protein: 30g

Turkey Meatloaf Muffins

Ingredients:

- pound lean ground turkey.
- 1/2 cup chopped onion.
- 1/4 cup mashed low-fiber vegetables (like zucchini or carrots)
- 1/4 cup low fiber breadcrumbs (like panko breadcrumbs)
- 1 egg, beaten.
- 1/4 cup low-fat milk
- 1 teaspoon dried oregano
- 1/4 teaspoon salt
- 1/4 teaspoon black pepper

Preparation Method:

- Preheat oven to 375°F (190°C). Use cooking spray to grease a 12-cup muffin pan.
- In a large bowl, combine ground turkey, onion, mashed vegetables, breadcrumbs, egg, milk, oregano, salt, and pepper. Mix well.
- Using muffin cups that have been prepped, divide the mixture equally.
- Bake for 20-25 minutes, or until cooked through (internal temperature reaches 165°F).
- Let cool slightly before serving.

Cooking Time: 20-25 minutes

Total Preparation Time: 30 minutes

Nutrition Value per serving (approximate):
Calories: 200
Fat: 8g

Carbohydrates: 15g
Protein: 20g

Poached Fish with Lemon-Herb Sauce

Ingredients:

- 2 skinless, boneless fish fillets (cod, tilapia, etc.)
- 2 cups low-sodium chicken broth
- 1 lemon, sliced.
- 2 sprigs fresh thyme or parsley
- Salt and black pepper to taste
- 1 tablespoon chopped fresh herbs (dill, parsley, or chives)
- 1 tablespoon low-fat yogurt (optional)

Preparation Method:

- Place fish fillets in a shallow pan or skillet. Add chicken broth, lemon slices, and thyme or parsley sprigs. Season with salt and pepper to taste.
- Bring to a simmer over medium heat. Cover and cook for 8-10 minutes, or until fish is cooked through and flakes easily with a fork.
- Remove fish from the pan and set aside on a plate.
- Strain the cooking broth into a small saucepan. Discard the lemon slices and herbs.
- (Optional) To thicken the sauce slightly, whisk in 1 tablespoon of low-fat yogurt.
- Simmer the sauce for a few minutes, until slightly reduced.
- Stir in chopped fresh herbs of your choice.
- Serve fish fillets with the lemon-herb sauce spooned over top.

Cooking Time: 8-10 minutes

Total Preparation Time: 15 minutes

Nutrition Value per serving (approximate):
Calories: 250
Fat: 5g
Carbohydrates: 5g

Protein: 40g

Scrambled Eggs with Mashed Avocado

Ingredients:

- 2 large eggs

- 1 tablespoon low-fat milk or water

- 1/2 ripe avocado

- 1 tablespoon olive oil (optional)

- Salt and pepper to taste

- Toast or crackers (optional)

Preparation Method:

- Crack the eggs into a bowl and whisk them together with the milk or water. Add a dash of pepper and salt for seasoning.

- Heat a non-stick pan over medium heat. If using oil, add a drizzle of olive oil and swirl to coat the pan.

- Pour the egg mixture into the pan and let it cook undisturbed for a minute.

- Gently stir the eggs with a spatula, allowing the uncooked portions to flow to the bottom of the pan. Continue to cook, stirring occasionally, until the eggs are just set but still slightly moist.

- While the eggs are cooking, mash the avocado with a fork in a separate bowl. Add a dash of salt and pepper for seasoning (optional).

- To serve, spoon the scrambled eggs onto a plate. Top with the mashed avocado.

- Optional: Serve with a slice of toast or crackers for dipping.

Cooking Time: 3-5 minutes

Total Preparation Time: 5-10 minutes

Portion Size: 1 serving.

Nutrition Value (approximate):
Calories: 250-300
Protein: 12-14 grams

Fat: 15-20 grams (depending on oil use)
Carbohydrates: 5-7 grams

Chicken and Vegetable Stir-Fry

Ingredients:

- One-pound chicken breast, thinly sliced, without bones and skin.
- 1 tablespoon low-sodium soy sauce
- 1 tablespoon cornstarch
- 1 tablespoon olive oil
- 1 cup chopped vegetables (broccoli florets, carrots, bell peppers, etc.) - well-cooked (can be steamed beforehand)
- 1/2 cup cooked white rice.
- Salt and pepper to taste

Preparation Method:

- Marinate the chicken: In a bowl, combine the sliced chicken breast with soy sauce and cornstarch. Give it a minimum of ten minutes to marinate.
- A wok or large pan should be heated to medium-high heat. To coat the pan, add the olive oil and swirl.
- Add the chicken to the pan and cook for 3-4 minutes, stirring frequently, until browned and cooked through.
- Add the well-cooked vegetables to the pan and stir-fry for another 1-2 minutes.
- Season with salt and pepper to taste.
- Add the cooked white rice to the pan and stir-fry for another minute to heat through.

Cooking Time: 8-10 minutes

Total Preparation Time: 15-20 minutes (including marinating time)

Portion Size: 1 serving.

Nutrition Value (approximate):
Calories: 400-450
Protein: 30-35 grams

Fat: 10-15 grams

Carbohydrates: 40-45 grams (depending on vegetables used)

Seafood Selections for Gastroparesis-Friendly Dinners:

Salmon with Creamy Dill Sauce:

Ingredients:

- 4 salmon fillets
- 1 tablespoon olive oil
- Salt and pepper to taste
- 1/4 cup Greek yogurt
- 2 tablespoons mayonnaise
- 1 tablespoon chopped fresh dill.
- 1 tablespoon lemon juice
- 1 teaspoon Dijon mustard

Preparation Method:

- Preheat the oven to 400°F (200°C).
- Season the salmon fillets with salt, pepper, and olive oil.
- The salmon should be cooked through after 12 to 15 minutes of baking it on a baking pan.
- In a small bowl, mix Greek yogurt, mayonnaise, chopped dill, lemon juice, and Dijon mustard to make the creamy dill sauce.
- Serve the baked salmon with the creamy dill sauce drizzled on top.

Cooking Time: 12-15 minutes

Total Preparation Time: 20 minutes

Portion Size: 1 salmon fillet.

Nutrition Value (per serving):
Calories: Approximately 300-350 kcal
Protein: Approximately 30-35g
Fat: Approximately 18-22g

Carbohydrates: Approximately 2-4g

Shrimp Scampi with Pasta:

Ingredients:

- 1 pound shrimp peeled and deveined.
- 8 ounces linguine pasta
- 3 tablespoons butter
- 3 cloves garlic, minced.
- 1/4 cup white wine
- 1/4 cup chicken broth
- Juice of 1 lemon
- Salt and pepper to taste
- Fresh parsley for garnish

Preparation Method:

- Linguine pasta should be cooked as directed on the package until it is al dente. After draining, set away.
- Heat a large skillet over medium heat to melt the butter. Cook the minced garlic for one to two minutes, or until it becomes aromatic.
- When the shrimp are pink and fully cooked, add them to the skillet and cook for two to three minutes on each side.
- Use chicken stock and white wine to deglaze the skillet. Add the lemon juice and salt and pepper to taste.
- Add the cooked pasta to the skillet and toss to coat with the shrimp and sauce.
- Serve the shrimp scampi with pasta garnished with fresh parsley.

Cooking Time: 15 minutes

Total Preparation Time: 25 minutes

Portion Size: Approximately 1/4 of the recipe.

Nutrition Value (per serving):

Calories: Approximately 400-450 kcal

| Protein: Approximately 25-30g |
| Fat: Approximately 15-20g |
| Carbohydrates: Approximately 35-40g |

Creamy Cod Chowder:

Ingredients:

- One-pound fish fillets, sliced into little pieces.
- 1 tablespoon olive oil
- 1 onion, diced.
- 2 carrots, diced.
- 2 celery stalks, diced.
- 3 cloves garlic, minced.
- 4 cups chicken or vegetable broth
- 1 cup diced potatoes.
- 1 bay leaf
- 1 cup heavy cream
- Salt and pepper to taste
- Chopped fresh parsley for garnish.

Preparation Method:

- Warm up the olive oil in a big pot over medium heat. Cook the diced onion, carrots, and celery for approximately five minutes, or until they become tender.
- When aromatic, add the minced garlic and simmer for one more minute.
- Pour in chicken or vegetable broth and bring to a simmer.
- Add diced potatoes and bay leaf to the pot. Simmer the potatoes for 10 to 12 minutes, or until they are soft.
- Stir in cod pieces and cook for 5-6 minutes until fish is cooked through.
- Remove the bay leaf from the chowder and stir in heavy cream. Season with salt and pepper to taste.
- Serve the creamy cod chowder garnished with chopped fresh parsley.

Cooking Time: Approximately 25 minutes

Total Preparation Time: 35 minutes

Portion Size: Approximately 1/4 of the recipe.

Nutrition Value (per serving):
Calories: Approximately 350-400 kcal
Protein: Approximately 20-25g
Fat: Approximately 20-25g
Carbohydrates: Approximately 15-20g

Tuna Salad on Crackers:

Ingredients:

- 2 cans (5 ounces each) tuna, drained.
- 1/4 cup mayonnaise
- 2 tablespoons diced celery.
- 2 tablespoons diced red onion.
- 1 tablespoon lemon juice
- Salt and pepper to taste
- Crackers for serving.
- Optional toppings: lettuce leaves, sliced tomatoes, avocado slices

Preparation Method:

- In a mixing bowl, combine drained tuna, mayonnaise, diced celery, diced red onion, and lemon juice. Mix well to combine.
- To taste, add more salt and pepper to the tuna salad.
- Top the tuna salad with crackers and serve.
- Optional: Serve with lettuce leaves, sliced tomatoes, and avocado slices for added freshness and flavor.

Portion Size: Approximately 1/4 of the recipe.

Nutrition Value (per serving, excluding crackers and optional toppings):
Calories: Approximately 150-200 kcal

Protein: Approximately 15-20g
Fat: Approximately 10-15g
Carbohydrates: Approximately 1-2g

Poached Tilapia with Lemon and Capers:

Ingredients:

- 4 tilapia fillets
- 2 tablespoons olive oil
- 1 lemon, sliced.
- 2 tablespoons capers
- Salt and pepper to taste
- Chopped fresh parsley for garnish.

Preparation Method:

- Season tilapia fillets with salt and pepper on both sides.
- Olive oil should be heated over medium heat in a big skillet. Add tilapia fillets and lemon slices to the skillet.
- Cook the tilapia for 3-4 minutes per side until cooked through.
- Remove the tilapia from the skillet and transfer to a serving dish.
- Sprinkle capers over the tilapia fillets and garnish with chopped fresh parsley.
- Serve the poached tilapia with lemon and capers immediately.

Cooking Time: Approximately 10 minutes

Total Preparation Time: 15 minutes

Portion Size: 1 tilapia fillet.

Nutrition Value (per serving):
Calories: Approximately 150-200 kcal
Protein: Approximately 20-25g
Fat: Approximately 8-10g
Carbohydrates: Approximately 1-2g

Creamy Tomato Pasta with Spinach:

Ingredients:

- 8 oz (225g) pasta of choice
- 1 tablespoon olive oil
- 2 cloves garlic, minced.
- 1 can (14 oz) diced tomatoes.
- 1/2 cup heavy cream
- 2 cups fresh spinach leaves
- Salt and pepper to taste
- Grated Parmesan cheese for serving (optional)

Preparation Method:

- Pasta should be cooked as directed on the package until it is al dente. After draining, set away.
- Heat the olive oil in a big skillet over medium heat. Add the minced garlic and simmer for one minute, or until fragrant.
- Stir in diced tomatoes (with juices) and cook for 5 minutes, until heated through.
- Add heavy cream and spinach to the skillet. Cook, stirring occasionally, until spinach wilts and the sauce thickens slightly, about 3-4 minutes.
- Season with salt and pepper to taste.
- When the pasta is ready, add it to the skillet and toss to uniformly coat it in sauce.
- If preferred, top the heated dish with grated Parmesan cheese.

Cooking Time: 15 minutes

Total Preparation Time: 25 minutes

Portion Size: 4 servings.

Nutrition Value (per serving):
Calories: Approximately 400 kcal
Protein: Approximately 10g

Fat: Approximately 15g
Carbohydrates: Approximately 55g
Fiber: Approximately 4g

Tofu Scramble with Vegetables:

Ingredients:

- Drained and crumbled one block (fourteen ounces) of firm tofu.
- 1 tablespoon olive oil
- 1 small onion, diced.
- 1 bell pepper, diced.
- 1 cup mushrooms, sliced.
- 2 cups spinach leaves
- 2 tablespoons nutritional yeast
- Salt and pepper to taste
- Fresh herbs for garnish (optional)

Preparation Method:

- Over medium heat, warm up the olive oil in a big skillet. Cook the chopped onion for three minutes, or until it becomes tender.
- Add sliced mushrooms and diced bell pepper to the skillet. Simmer for 5 minutes or until veggies are soft.
- Stir in crumbled tofu and nutritional yeast. Cook, stirring occasionally, until tofu is heated through and slightly browned, about 5 minutes.
- Add spinach leaves to the skillet and cook until wilted, about 2 minutes.
- Season with salt and pepper to taste. Garnish with fresh herbs if desired.
- Serve hot as a breakfast or brunch option.

Cooking Time: 15 minutes

Total Preparation Time: 25 minutes

Portion Size: 4 servings.

Nutrition Value (per serving):

Calories: Approximately 150 kcal
Protein: Approximately 12g
Fat: Approximately 8g
Carbohydrates: Approximately 10g
Fiber: Approximately 4g

Vegetable Egg Bake:

Ingredients:

- 8 eggs
- 1/4 cup milk (or dairy-free alternative)
- 1 cup diced bell peppers.
- 1 cup diced zucchini.
- 1 cup diced tomatoes.
- 1 cup spinach leaves
- Salt and pepper to taste
- Grated cheese for topping (optional)

Preparation Method:

- Preheat the oven to 350°F (175°C). Apply cooking spray or olive oil to a baking dish to grease it.
- In a large mixing bowl, whisk together eggs and milk until well combined.
- Stir in diced bell peppers, zucchini, tomatoes, and spinach leaves. Season with salt and pepper to taste.
- Fill the baking dish with the egg mixture.
- Bake for 25 to 30 minutes in a preheated oven, or until the tops of the eggs are gently brown and set.
- Take out of the oven and allow it to cool down a little before slicing.
- Serve hot, topped with grated cheese if desired.

Cooking Time: 30 minutes

Total Preparation Time: 40 minutes

Portion Size: 6 servings.

Nutrition Value (per serving):
Calories: Approximately 150 kcal
Protein: Approximately 12g
Fat: Approximately 8g
Carbohydrates: Approximately 8g
Fiber: Approximately 2g

Creamy Mashed Potato and Butternut Squash:

Ingredients:

- 2 cups peeled and cubed butternut squash.
- 2 cups peeled and cubed potatoes.
- 2 tablespoons butter (or dairy-free alternative)
- 1/4 cup milk (or dairy-free alternative)
- Salt and pepper to taste
- Fresh herbs for garnish (optional)

Preparation Method:

- Place cubed butternut squash and potatoes in a large pot. Bring the water to a boil while covering.
- Reduce heat to medium and simmer for 15-20 minutes, or until vegetables are tender when pierced with a fork.
- Drain the cooked vegetables and return them to the pot.
- Add butter and milk to the pot. Use a potato masher or fork to mash the vegetables until smooth and creamy.
- Season with salt and pepper to taste. Garnish with fresh herbs if desired.
- Serve hot as a comforting side dish.

Cooking Time: 25 minutes

Total Preparation Time: 35 minutes

Portion Size: 4 servings.

Nutrition Value (per serving):
Calories: Approximately 150 kcal
Protein: Approximately 2g
Fat: Approximately 6g
Carbohydrates: Approximately 25g
Fiber: Approximately 4g

Avocado Toast with Scrambled Eggs and Tomato:

Ingredients:

- 4 slices whole grain bread (gluten-free if needed)
- 1 ripe avocado
- 4 eggs
- 1 tomato, sliced.
- Salt and pepper to taste
- Fresh herbs for garnish (optional)

Preparation Method:

- Toast the whole grain bread pieces till they are golden and crunchy.
- While the bread is toasting, prepare the scrambled eggs. In a skillet, scramble the eggs over medium heat until cooked through. Season with salt and pepper, to taste.
- Squash the ripe avocado in a little dish.
- Spread mashed avocado evenly onto each slice of toasted bread.
- Top the avocado toast with scrambled eggs and sliced tomato.
- Garnish with fresh herbs if desired.

Cooking Time: 15 minutes

Total Preparation Time: 20 minutes

Portion Size: 4 servings.

Nutrition Value (per serving):
Calories: Approximately 250 kcal

Protein: Approximately 12g
Fat: Approximately 12g
Carbohydrates: Approximately 25g
Fiber: Approximately 8g

Comforting Casseroles and One-Pot Meals:

Chicken and Rice Casserole:

Ingredients:

- 2 cups cooked chicken, shredded, or diced.

- 1 cup uncooked white rice

- 2 cups chicken broth

- 1 cup frozen mixed vegetables

- 1 cup shredded cheddar cheese

- 1 teaspoon garlic powder

- Salt and pepper to taste

Preparation Method:

- Preheat the oven to 375°F (190°C).

- In a casserole dish, combine the cooked chicken, uncooked rice, chicken broth, frozen mixed vegetables, shredded cheddar cheese, garlic powder, salt, and pepper. Mix well.

- Cover the casserole dish with foil and bake for 45-50 minutes or until the rice is cooked and the liquid is absorbed.

- Take it out of the oven, let it a few minutes to cool, and then serve.

Cooking Time: 45-50 minutes

Total Preparation Time: Approximately 1 hour

Portion Size: 1 cup.

Nutrition Value (per serving):
Calories: 350
Protein: 25g
Carbohydrates: 35g
Fat: 12g
Fiber: 3g

<u>Tuna Noodle Casserole:</u>

Ingredients:

- 8 oz (225g) egg noodles, cooked according to package instructions.

- 2 cans (5 oz each) tuna, drained.

- 1 cup frozen peas

- One can (10.5 oz) of cream of mushroom soup

- 1 cup shredded cheddar cheese

- 1 teaspoon garlic powder

- Salt and pepper to taste

- Crushed potato chips for topping (optional)

Preparation Method:

- Preheat the oven to 375°F (190°C).

- In a large bowl, combine the cooked egg noodles, drained tuna, frozen peas, cream of mushroom soup, shredded cheddar cheese, garlic powder, salt, and pepper. Mix well.

- Transfer the mixture to a casserole dish. If desired, sprinkle crumbled potato chips on top.

- Bake for 25 to 30 minutes, or until the tops are bubbly and brown.

- Take it out of the oven, let it a few minutes to cool, and then serve.

Cooking Time: 25-30 minutes

Total Preparation Time: Approximately 45 minutes

Portion Size: 1 cup.

Nutrition Value (per serving):
Calories: 400
Protein: 25g
Carbohydrates: 30g
Fat: 20g
Fiber: 3g

Cheesy Eggplant Parmesan:

Ingredients:

- 1 large eggplant, sliced into 1/2-inch rounds.

- 1 cup marinara sauce

- 1 cup shredded mozzarella cheese

- 1/4 cup grated Parmesan cheese.

- 1/2 cup breadcrumbs (gluten-free if desired)

- 1 teaspoon Italian seasoning

- Salt and pepper to taste

- Olive oil for brushing

Preparation Method:

- Preheat the oven to 400°F (200°C).

- Brush both sides of the eggplant slices with olive oil and season with salt and pepper. Place them on a baking sheet and bake for 15-20 minutes or until tender.

- In a small bowl, mix the breadcrumbs and Italian seasoning.

- In a greased baking dish, layer the baked eggplant slices with marinara sauce, shredded mozzarella cheese, grated Parmesan cheese, and breadcrumb mixture.

- Layers should be repeated until all ingredients have been used, and then topped with a layer of cheese and breadcrumbs.

- Bake the cheese for 25 to 30 minutes, or until it is bubbling and melted.

- Take it out of the oven, let it a few minutes to cool, and then serve.

Cooking Time: 40-50 minutes

Total Preparation Time: Approximately 1 hour

Portion Size: 1 slice.

Nutrition Value (per serving):
Calories: 250
Protein: 10g
Carbohydrates: 20g
Fat: 15g
Fiber: 5g

<u>One-Pot Creamy Tomato Chicken:</u>

Ingredients:

- 4 boneless, skinless chicken breasts

- 1 tablespoon olive oil

- 1 onion, diced.

- 2 cloves garlic, minced.

- 1 can (14 oz) diced tomatoes.

- 1 cup chicken broth

- 1/2 cup heavy cream

- 1 teaspoon Italian seasoning

- Salt and pepper to taste

- Fresh basil leaves for garnish (optional)

Preparation Method:

- Add salt, pepper, and Italian seasoning to the chicken breasts.

- Heat the olive oil in a big saucepan or skillet over medium heat. After adding the chicken breasts, sear them for about 5 minutes on each side, or until browned all over. Take out of the skillet and place it aside.

- Add the chopped onion and minced garlic to the same skillet. Cook until softened, about 3-4 minutes.

- Add the diced tomatoes (with juices) and chicken broth to the skillet. Bring to a simmer.

- Return the chicken breasts to the skillet and simmer for 15-20 minutes or until the chicken is cooked through.

- Cook for a further five minutes after stirring in the heavy cream.

- Serve immediately, garnishing with fresh basil leaves if preferred.

Cooking Time: 35-40 minutes

Total Preparation Time: Approximately 50 minutes

Portion Size: 1 chicken breast with sauce.

Nutrition Value (per serving):
Calories: 300
Protein: 30g
Carbohydrates: 10g
Fat: 15g
Fiber: 2g

<u>Turkey Shepherd's Pie:</u>

Ingredients:

- 1 lb. ground turkey

- 1 onion, diced.

- 2 cloves garlic, minced.

- 2 cups frozen mixed vegetables

- 1 cup chicken broth

- 2 tablespoons tomato paste

- 2 cups mashed potatoes.

- 1/2 cup shredded cheddar cheese

- Salt and pepper to taste

Preparation Method:

- Preheat the oven to 375°F (190°C).

- The ground turkey should be cooked in a large skillet over medium heat. Cook the minced garlic and chopped onion until they are tender.

- Stir in the frozen mixed vegetables, chicken broth, and tomato paste. Season with salt and pepper to taste. Simmer for 10-15 minutes.

- Pour the mixture of turkey into a baking dish that has been oiled. On top, distribute the mashed potatoes.

- Over the mashed potatoes, evenly distribute the shredded cheddar cheese.

- Bake the cheese for 25 to 30 minutes, or until it is bubbling and melted.

- Take it out of the oven, let it a few minutes to cool, and then serve.

Cooking Time: 40-45 minutes

Total Preparation Time: Approximately 1 hour

Portion Size: 1 slice.

Nutrition Value (per serving):
Calories: 350
Protein: 20g
Carbohydrates: 25g
Fat: 18g
Fiber: 4g

Snacks and Small Bites

Creamy Yogurt with Applesauce:

Ingredients:

- Low-fat yogurt
- Unsweetened applesauce

Preparation Method:

- In a bowl, combine the desired amount of low-fat yogurt with an equal amount of unsweetened applesauce.
- Mix well until smooth and creamy.

Total Preparation Time: 5 minutes

Portion Size: 1 serving.

Nutrition Value (per serving):
Calories: Varies based on portion size
Protein: Varies based on yogurt
Fat: Varies based on yogurt
Carbohydrates: Varies based on yogurt and applesauce
Fiber: Varies based on yogurt and applesauce
Sugar: Varies based on yogurt and applesauce

Smashed Avocado on Crackers:

Ingredients:

- Ripe avocado
- Crackers (choose gluten-free if desired)

Preparation Method:

- Scoop out the flesh from the ripe avocado into a bowl after cutting it in half and removing the pit.
- Using a fork, mash the avocado until it has the consistency you want.
- Spread the mashed avocado onto crackers.

Total Preparation Time: 5 minutes

Portion Size: 1 serving.

Nutrition Value (per serving):
Calories: Varies based on portion size and type of crackers
Protein: Varies based on portion size
Fat: Varies based on portion size and avocado
Carbohydrates: Varies based on portion size and crackers
Fiber: Varies based on portion size and crackers
Sugar: Minimal, primarily from crackers

Scrambled Egg Bites:

Ingredients:

- Eggs
- Low-fat milk (optional)
- Chopped vegetables (e.g., spinach, bell peppers)
- Salt and pepper to taste

Preparation Method:

- In a bowl, whisk together eggs and a splash of low-fat milk (if desired).
- Stir in chopped vegetables, salt, and pepper.
- Pour the mixture into a greased muffin tin, filling each cup about halfway.
- Bake in a preheated oven at 350°F (175°C) for 15-20 minutes or until the eggs are set.

Cooking Time: 15-20 minutes

Total Preparation Time: 25-30 minutes

Portion Size: 1-2 egg bites per serving.

Nutrition Value (per serving):
Calories: Varies based on portion size and ingredients
Protein: Varies based on portion size and eggs
Fat: Varies based on portion size and ingredients
Carbohydrates: Varies based on portion size and vegetables

Fiber: Varies based on portion size and vegetables
Sugar: Minimal, primarily from vegetables

Banana with Nut Butter:

Ingredients:

- Ripe banana
- Nut butter (e.g., peanut butter, almond butter)

Preparation Method:

- Peel the ripe banana and slice it into rounds.
- Spread nut butter onto each banana slice.

Total Preparation Time: 5 minutes

Portion Size: 1 serving.

Nutrition Value (per serving):
Calories: Varies based on portion size and type of nut butter
Protein: Varies based on portion size and nut butter
Fat: Varies based on portion size and nut butter
Carbohydrates: Varies based on portion size and banana
Fiber: Varies based on portion size and banana
Sugar: Minimal, primarily from banana

Cantaloupe with Cottage Cheese:

Ingredients:

- Cantaloupe
- Cottage cheese (low-fat if desired)

Preparation Method:

- Cut the cantaloupe in half, remove the seeds, and slice into wedges or cubes.
- Serve with a dollop of cottage cheese on top or on the side.

Total Preparation Time: 5 minutes

Portion Size: 1 serving.

Nutrition Value (per serving):
Calories: Varies based on portion size and type of cottage cheese
Protein: Varies based on portion size and cottage cheese
Fat: Varies based on portion size and cottage cheese
Carbohydrates: Varies based on portion size and cantaloupe
Fiber: Varies based on portion size and cantaloupe
Sugar: Minimal, primarily from cantaloupe

Hard-Boiled Eggs

Ingredients:

- Eggs
- Water

Preparation Method:

- Transfer the eggs to the bottom of a saucepan in a single layer.
- Make sure the eggs are at least an inch under the cold water by covering them with it.
- Put the water on medium-high heat and bring it to a boil.
- Once boiling, remove the saucepan from the heat and cover it with a lid.
- Let the eggs sit in the hot water for 10-12 minutes for medium-sized eggs (adjust time for larger or smaller eggs).
- After the desired cooking time, transfer the eggs to a bowl of ice water to cool for a few minutes.
- Peel the eggs under cool running water and pat dry with paper towels.

Cooking Time: 10-12 minutes

Total Preparation Time: Approximately 15 minutes

Portion Size: Typically, 1-2 eggs per serving.

Nutrition Value (per serving):
Calories: Approximately 70-80 kcal per egg

Protein: Approximately 6 grams per egg
Fat: Approximately 5 grams per egg
Carbohydrates: Approximately 0 grams per egg
Other nutrients: Eggs are rich in vitamins and minerals, including vitamin D, vitamin B12, selenium, and choline.

<u>Yogurt with Trail Mix (Limited Nuts and Seeds)</u>

Ingredients:

- Plain low-fat yogurt
- Trail mix (containing limited nuts and seeds)
- Optional: honey or maple syrup for sweetness

Preparation Method:

- Scoop desired amount of plain low-fat yogurt into a serving bowl.
- Top the yogurt with a portion of trail mix, ensuring it contains limited nuts and seeds to maintain digestibility.
- Drizzle with honey or maple syrup if desired for sweetness.

Total Preparation Time: Approximately 5 minutes

Portion Size: 1 serving.

Nutrition Value (per serving):
Calories: Varies depending on yogurt and trail mix brands
Protein: Varies depending on yogurt and trail mix brands
Fat: Varies depending on yogurt and trail mix brands
Carbohydrates: Varies depending on yogurt and trail mix brands
Other nutrients: Provides protein, healthy fats, and carbohydrates, along with vitamins and minerals from yogurt and trail mix ingredients.

<u>Strained Fruit or Vegetable Juice</u>

Ingredients:

- Fresh fruits or vegetables (e.g., apples, carrots, cucumbers)

- Water (if needed for blending)

- Optional: lemon juice or ginger for flavor

Preparation Method:

- Wash and chop the fruits or vegetables into small pieces.

- Place the chopped ingredients in a blender or food processor.

- Blend until smooth.

- Strain the mixture through a fine-mesh sieve or cheesecloth to remove pulp and fiber.

- Add lemon juice or ginger for additional flavor if desired.

- Serve chilled or over ice.

Total Preparation Time: Approximately 10-15 minutes

Portion Size: 1 serving.

Nutrition Value (per serving):
Calories: Varies depending on fruits or vegetables used
Fiber: Minimal, as the juice is strained
Vitamins and minerals: Provides vitamins and minerals present in the fruits or vegetables used.

Sliced Apples and Low-Fat Cheese

Ingredients:

- Apples
- Low-fat cheese slices or cubes

Preparation Method:

- Wash and slice the apples into thin wedges or rounds.
- Arrange the sliced apples on a plate.
- Serve with low-fat cheese slices or cubes.

Total Preparation Time: Approximately 5 minutes

Portion Size: 1 serving.

Nutrition Value (per serving):
Calories: Varies depending on the type and amount of cheese used
Protein: Varies depending on the type and amount of cheese used
Fat: Varies depending on the type and amount of cheese used
Carbohydrates: Varies depending on the number of apples and type of cheese used

Other nutrients: Provides vitamins and minerals from apples and cheese, along with protein and calcium from cheese.

Rice Cakes with Mashed Avocado

Ingredients:

- Rice cakes
- Ripe avocados

Preparation Method:

- Peel and pit the ripe avocados.
- In a bowl, mash the avocados with a fork until smooth.
- Spread the mashed avocado onto rice cakes.

Total Preparation Time: Approximately 5 minutes
Portion Size: 1 serving.

Nutrition Value (per serving):
Calories: Varies depending on the size of rice cakes and amount of avocado used
Protein: Varies depending on the amount of avocado used
Fat: Varies depending on the amount of avocado used
Carbohydrates: Varies depending on the size of rice cakes and amount of avocado used
Other nutrients: Provides healthy fats, fiber, and various vitamins and minerals from avocados. Rice cakes contribute minimal fat and calories.

Sweet Treats and Desserts

Creamy Banana Popsicles:

Ingredients:

- Ripe bananas
- Greek yogurt (or dairy-free yogurt alternative)
- Honey or maple syrup (optional)
- Vanilla extract (optional)

Preparation Method:

- Peel the bananas and cut them into chunks.
- Blend the banana chunks with Greek yogurt until smooth. Add honey or maple syrup and vanilla extract if desired.
- Pour the mixture into popsicle molds.
- Insert popsicle sticks into each mold.
- Freeze until solid, preferably for 4 hours.

Cooking Time: None (Freezing time required)

Total Preparation Time: 10 minutes (plus freezing time)

Portion Size: Depends on the size of the popsicle molds.

Nutrition Value:

Creamy banana popsicles are typically low in calories and fat. They provide potassium from the bananas and protein from the yogurt. The nutrition content may vary based on specific ingredients and portion sizes.

Baked Apples with Cinnamon:

Ingredients:

- Apples (preferably firm varieties like Granny Smith)
- Ground cinnamon.
- Honey or maple syrup (optional)
- Chopped nuts (optional)

Preparation Method:

- Preheat the oven to 375°F (190°C).
- Core the apples, leaving the bottom intact.
- Place the apples in a baking dish.
- If preferred, drizzle honey or maple syrup over the apples after they have been sprinkled with cinnamon.
- Bake for twenty to thirty minutes, or until apples are soft.
- Serve warm, optionally topped with chopped nuts.

Cooking Time: 25-30 minutes

Total Preparation Time: 35-40 minutes

Portion Size: 1 baked apple per serving.

Nutrition Value:
Baked apples with cinnamon are low in calories and fat. They provide fiber from the apples and can be a source of natural sweetness without added sugars if no sweeteners are used.

Cantaloupe and Honeydew Skewers with Yogurt Dip:

Ingredients:

- Cantaloupe, cubed.
- Honeydew melon, cubed.
- Wooden skewers
- Greek yogurt (or dairy-free yogurt alternative)
- Honey
- Fresh mint leaves (optional, for garnish)

Preparation Method:

- Thread alternating pieces of cantaloupe and honeydew onto wooden skewers.
- In a small bowl, mix Greek yogurt with honey to taste for the dip.
- Serve the skewers with the yogurt dip.
- Garnish with fresh mint leaves if desired.

Cooking Time: None

Total Preparation Time: 15 minutes

Portion Size: Depends on the number of skewers prepared.

Skinny Rice Pudding:

Ingredients:

- Cooked white rice.
- Almond milk (or any milk of choice)
- Maple syrup or honey
- Vanilla extract
- Ground cinnamon.
- Raisins or dried cranberries (optional)

Preparation Method:

- In a saucepan, combine cooked rice and almond milk.
- Stirring regularly, cook the mixture over medium heat until it thickens.
- Stir in maple syrup or honey, vanilla extract, and ground cinnamon to taste.
- Continue cooking for a few more minutes until the pudding reaches the desired consistency.
- Remove from heat and let cool.
- Serve chilled or at room temperature, optionally topped with raisins or dried cranberries.

Cooking Time: 20-25 minutes

Total Preparation Time: 30-35 minutes

Portion Size: Depends on serving size preference.

Nutrition Value:

Skinny rice pudding made with almond milk and sweetened with natural sweeteners is lower in calories and fat compared to traditional rice pudding recipes. It provides carbohydrates from the rice and almond milk and can be a good source of calcium and vitamins.

Avocado Chocolate Mousse:

Ingredients:

- Ripe avocados
- Unsweetened cocoa powder
- Honey or maple syrup
- Vanilla extract
- Almond milk or any milk of choice

Preparation Method:

- Remove the ripe avocado flesh and place it in a food processor or blender.
- Add cocoa powder, honey or maple syrup, and vanilla extract to taste.
- Blend until smooth, adding almond milk as needed to achieve the desired consistency.
- Spoon the mixture into glasses or serving dishes.
- Before serving, let the food cool for at least half an hour in the refrigerator.

Total Preparation Time: 10 minutes (plus chilling time)

Portion Size: Depends on serving size preference.

Nutrition Value:

Avocado chocolate mousse is rich in heart-healthy fats from avocados and antioxidants from cocoa powder. It's lower in sugar compared to traditional chocolate mousse recipes, especially if sweetened with honey or maple syrup.

Peach Melba with a Twist:

Ingredients:

- 2 ripe peaches, sliced.
- 1/2 cup raspberries
- 1 tablespoon honey
- 1/4 cup low-fat Greek yogurt
- 1 tablespoon chopped almonds.

Preparation Method:

- Arrange peach slices and raspberries on a serving plate.
- Drizzle honey over the fruit.
- Top with a dollop of Greek yogurt.
- Sprinkle chopped almonds on top.

Cooking Time: None

Total Preparation Time: 5 minutes

Portion Size: 1 serving.

Nutrition Value (per serving):
Calories: 150
Protein: 5g
Carbohydrates: 25g
Fat: 4g
Fiber: 5g

Creamy Mango Lassi:

Ingredients:

- 1 ripe mango peeled and chopped.
- 1/2 cup low-fat Greek yogurt
- 1/4 cup low-fat milk
- 1 tablespoon honey (optional)
- 1/4 teaspoon ground cardamom (optional)

Preparation Method:

- Place chopped mango, Greek yogurt, milk, honey (if using), and cardamom (if using) in a blender.
- Blend until smooth and creamy.
- Serve chilled.

Total Preparation Time: 5 minutes

Portion Size: 1 serving.

Nutrition Value (per serving):
Calories: 180
Protein: 8g
Carbohydrates: 30g
Fat: 3g
Fiber: 3g

Frozen Yogurt Bark with Melba Toast:

Ingredients:

- 1 cup low-fat Greek yogurt
- 1 tablespoon honey
- 1/4 cup sliced strawberries.
- 1/4 cup blueberries

- 2 Melba toast crackers, crushed.

Preparation Method:

- Line a baking sheet with parchment paper.
- Greek yogurt and honey should be thoroughly mixed in a bowl.
- Spread the yogurt mixture evenly on the prepared baking sheet.
- Sprinkle sliced strawberries, blueberries, and crushed Melba toast on top.
- Freeze for 2-3 hours until firm.
- Break into pieces and serve as a frozen treat.

Cooking Time: 2-3 hours (freezing)

Total Preparation Time: 10 minutes (plus freezing time)

Portion Size: 4 servings.

Nutrition Value (per serving):
Calories: 70
Protein: 4g
Carbohydrates: 10g
Fat: 2g
Fiber: 1g

Banana Nut Butter Smoothie:

Ingredients:

- 1 ripe banana
- 2 tablespoons nut butter (peanut, almond, or cashew)
- 1/2 cup low-fat milk or almond milk
- 1/4 teaspoon ground cinnamon (optional)
- Ice cubes (optional)

Preparation Method:

- Place banana, nut butter, milk, and ground cinnamon (if using) in a blender.
- Add ice cubes if desired.
- Blend until smooth and creamy.
- Serve immediately.

Total Preparation Time: 5 minutes

Portion Size: 1 serving.

Nutrition Value (per serving):
Calories: 250
Protein: 8g
Carbohydrates: 30g

Fat: 12g
Fiber: 4g

Strained Fruit Punch:

Ingredients:

- 1 cup mixed fruit juice (strained to remove pulp)
- 1/2 cup sparkling water or club soda
- 1 tablespoon honey or agave syrup (optional)
- Ice cubes.
- Sliced fruits for garnish (optional)

Preparation Method:

- In a pitcher, mix mixed fruit juice, sparkling water, and honey or agave syrup (if using).
- Stir until well combined.
- Place in the fridge to chill until you're ready to serve.
- Serve over ice cubes and garnish with sliced fruits if desired.

Total Preparation Time: 5 minutes (plus chilling time)

Portion Size: 2 servings.

Nutrition Value (per serving):
Calories: 60
Protein: 0g
Carbohydrates: 15g
Fat: 0g
Fiber: 0g

SPECIAL DIETS AND CONSIDERATIONS

Gluten-Free and Dairy-Free Options

Tropical Smoothie:

Ingredients:

- 1 ripe banana peeled and sliced.
- 1/2 cup chopped cantaloupe.
- 1/2 cup low-sugar coconut milk
- Splash of water (optional)
- Ice cubes (optional)

Preparation Method:

- Place the sliced banana, chopped cantaloupe, and coconut milk in a blender.
- Blend until smooth. If the smoothie is too thick, add a splash of water to reach the desired consistency.
- If desired, add ice cubes and mix once more until smooth.
- Pour into glasses and serve immediately.

Total Preparation Time: 5 minutes

Portion Size: 1 serving.

Nutrition Value (per serving):
Calories: Approximately 180
Protein: 2g
Fat: 7g
Carbohydrates: 32g
Fiber: 3g
Sugars: 20g

Salmon with Coconut Rice and Steamed Veggies:

Ingredients:

- 2 salmon fillets

- 1 cup jasmine rice

- 1 cup low-fat coconut milk

- 1 cup water

- Assorted vegetables for steaming (e.g., broccoli, carrots, snow peas)

Preparation Method:

- Preheat the oven to 375°F (190°C).

- Season the salmon fillets with salt, pepper, and lemon pepper seasoning.

- Add the water, coconut milk, and jasmine rice to a saucepan. Bring to a boil, then reduce heat to low, cover, and simmer for 15-20 minutes, or until the rice is cooked and the liquid is absorbed.

- While the rice is cooking, place the seasoned salmon fillets on a baking sheet lined with parchment paper. Bake for 12 to 15 minutes, or until the salmon is cooked through, in an oven that has been warmed.

- Steam the assorted vegetables until tender, about 5-7 minutes.

- Serve the cooked salmon with coconut rice and steamed veggies.

Cooking Time: 12-15 minutes for salmon; 15-20 minutes for rice

Total Preparation Time: Approximately 35-40 minutes

Portion Size: 2 servings.

Nutrition Value (per serving):
Calories: Approximately 450
Protein: 30g
Fat: 20g
Carbohydrates: 35g
Fiber: 3g
Sugars: 1g (from coconut milk)

Tofu Scramble with Mashed Avocado:

Ingredients:

- 1 block firm tofu, crumbled.

- 1/2 tablespoon olive oil

- 1/4 cup chopped bell peppers.

- 1/4 cup chopped onions.

- 1/4 teaspoon turmeric

- 2 ripe avocados

- Salt and pepper to taste

Preparation Method:

- In a skillet over medium heat, warm the olive oil. Add chopped bell peppers and onions, and sauté until softened.

- Add crumbled tofu to the skillet and sprinkle with turmeric. Cook until thoroughly cooked and beginning to turn golden.

- In a separate bowl, mash the ripe avocados with a fork until smooth. Season with salt and pepper to taste.

- Serve the tofu scramble with mashed avocado on the side.

Cooking Time: 10-15 minutes

Total Preparation Time: Approximately 20 minutes

Portion Size: 2 servings.

Nutrition Value (per serving):
Calories: Approximately 320
Protein: 14g
Fat: 25g
Carbohydrates: 15g
Fiber: 9g
Sugars: 2g

Chicken Stir-Fry with Rice Noodles:

Ingredients:

- 2 boneless, skinless chicken breasts thinly sliced.

- 1 tablespoon olive oil

- 2 cups mixed vegetables (e.g., carrots, bell peppers, snap peas)

- 6 oz rice noodles, cooked according to package instructions.

- 2 tablespoons low-sodium soy sauce

- 1 tablespoon hoisin sauce

- 1 teaspoon sesame oil

- Garnish with chopped green onions and sesame seeds, if desired.

Preparation Method:

- In a big wok or skillet, warm up the olive oil over medium-high heat. Add sliced chicken breasts and cook until no longer pink, about 5-6 minutes.

- Add mixed vegetables to the skillet and stir-fry until tender-crisp, about 3–4 minutes.

- In a small bowl, whisk together soy sauce, hoisin sauce, and sesame oil. Drizzle the sauce over the veggies and chicken in the skillet.

- Add cooked rice noodles to the skillet and toss to combine, ensuring the noodles are evenly coated with the sauce.

- Cook for an additional 1-2 minutes, or until everything is heated through.

- If preferred, garnish with sesame seeds and chopped green onions. Serve hot.

Cooking Time: Approximately 15 minutes

Total Preparation Time: Approximately 25 minutes (excluding noodle cooking time)

Portion Size: 2 servings.

Nutrition Value (per serving):
Calories: Approximately 400
Protein: 30g
Fat: 10g
Carbohydrates: 45g
Fiber: 4g

Sugars: 5g

Tuna Salad on Rice Cakes:

Ingredients:

- One 5-ounce can (drained) of tuna in water
- 2 tablespoons low-fat mayonnaise
- 1 tablespoon chopped celery.
- 1 tablespoon chopped red onion.
- 1 tablespoon chopped pickles.
- Salt and pepper to taste
- 4 rice cakes

Preparation Method:

- In a mixing bowl, combine drained tuna, low-fat mayonnaise, chopped celery, chopped red onion, and chopped pickles. Mix well to combine.
- Add salt and pepper to taste when preparing the tuna salad.
- Divide the tuna salad evenly among the rice cakes, spreading it over the top of each rice cake.
- Serve right away or put in the fridge until you're ready to serve.

Total Preparation Time: Approximately 10 minutes

Portion Size: 2 servings (2 rice cakes per serving)

Nutrition Value (per serving):
Calories: Approximately 180
Protein: 15g
Fat: 5g
Carbohydrates: 20g
Fiber: 1g
Sugars: 1g

Scrambled Eggs with Spinach and Avocado:

Ingredients:

- 2 eggs
- 1 cup fresh spinach leaves
- 1/2 avocado, mashed.
- Salt and pepper to taste

Preparation Method:

- In a bowl, whisk together the eggs and add pepper and salt to taste.
- Place the spinach leaves in a nonstick skillet and cook it over medium heat. Sauté until wilted.
- Scramble the prepared eggs until fully cooked by pouring them over the spinach after whisking them.
- Serve the scrambled eggs topped with mashed avocado.

Cooking Time: 5 minutes

Total Preparation Time: 10 minutes

Portion Size: 1 serving.

Nutrition Value (per serving):
Calories: 280
Protein: 14g
Carbohydrates: 9g
Fat: 21g
Fiber: 5g

<u>**Poached Fish with Lemon-Herb Sauce:**</u>

Ingredients:

- 2 white fish fillets (such as cod or tilapia)

- 1 lemon, sliced.

- Fresh herbs (such as dill or parsley)

- Salt and pepper to taste

Preparation Method:

- Add salt and pepper to the fish fillets for seasoning.

- In a shallow pan, combine the fresh herbs and lemon segments.

- Place the fish fillets over the slices of lemon.

- Cover the pan and poach the fish over low heat until cooked through.

- Serve the poached fish with lemon slices and fresh herbs.

Cooking Time: 10 minutes

Total Preparation Time: 20 minutes

Portion Size: 1 serving.

Nutrition Value (per serving):
Calories: 200
Protein: 30g
Carbohydrates: 2g
Fat: 8g
Fiber: 1g

<u>White Bean and Vegetable Soup:</u>

Ingredients:

- 1 can white beans, drained and rinsed.

- 2 carrots, diced.

- 2 celery stalks, diced.

- 1 onion, diced.

- 2 cloves garlic, minced.

- 4 cups low-sodium vegetable broth
- Salt and pepper to taste

Preparation Method:

- In a big pot, warm up the olive oil over medium heat. Cook the celery, carrots, and onions until they are tender.
- Cook for a further minute after adding the minced garlic.
- After adding the vegetable broth, boil the mixture.
- Add the white beans to the pot and simmer for 15-20 minutes.
- Season with salt and pepper to taste.
- Serve hot.

Cooking Time: 25 minutes

Total Preparation Time: 35 minutes

Portion Size: 1 cup.

Nutrition Value (per serving):
Calories: 180
Protein: 8g
Carbohydrates: 30g
Fat: 2g
Fiber: 8g

Turkey and Veggie Meatloaf Muffins:

Ingredients:

- 1 lb. lean ground turkey
- 1 zucchini, grated.
- 1 carrot, grated.
- 1/2 onion finely chopped.
- 2 cloves garlic, minced.
- 1/4 cup almond flour
- 1 egg

- Salt and pepper to taste

Preparation Method:

- Preheat the oven to 375°F (190°C). Grease a muffin tin.
- In a large bowl, mix the ground turkey, grated zucchini, grated carrot, chopped onion, minced garlic, almond flour, egg, salt, and pepper.
- Evenly distribute the mixture among the muffin cups.
- Bake the meatloaf muffins for 25 to 30 minutes, or until they are thoroughly cooked.
- Let cool slightly before serving.

Cooking Time: 30 minutes

Total Preparation Time: 45 minutes

Portion Size: 2 muffins.

Nutrition Value (per serving):
Calories: 250
Protein: 25g
Carbohydrates: 10g
Fat: 12g
Fiber: 2g

<u>Chicken and Vegetable Stir-Fry with Brown Rice:</u>

Ingredients:

- 1 lb. chicken breast, sliced.
- Two cups of mixed veggies, including snap peas, broccoli, and bell peppers
- 2 cloves garlic, minced.
- 1 tablespoon ginger, minced.
- 2 tablespoons low-sodium soy sauce
- 1 tablespoon sesame oil
- Cooked brown rice, for serving.

Preparation Method:

- In a large skillet or wok, heat the sesame oil over medium-high heat.

- When the chicken breast is well cooked and browned, add it and slice it.
- Add the ginger and garlic, minced, and sauté for an additional one minute.
- Stir-fry the mixed vegetables in the skillet until they become crisp-tender.
- Add the low-sodium soy sauce and mix everything together.
- Over cooked brown rice, serve the stir-fried chicken and vegetables.

Cooking Time: 20 minutes

Total Preparation Time: 30 minutes

Portion Size: 1.5 cups.

Nutrition Value (per serving):
Calories: 300
Protein: 30g
Carbohydrates: 25g
Fat: 8g
Fiber: 5g

Vegetarian and Vegan Adaptations:

Lentil Soup with Vegetables:

Ingredients:

- 1 cup dried lentils
- 4 cups low-sodium vegetable broth
- 1 onion, chopped.
- 2 carrots, diced.
- 2 celery stalks, diced.
- 1 can diced tomatoes.
- 2 cloves garlic, minced.

- 1 teaspoon dried thyme

- Salt and pepper to taste

Preparation Method:

- Rinse the lentils under cold water.

- In a large pot, combine the lentils, vegetable broth, onion, carrots, celery, diced tomatoes, garlic, and dried thyme.

- Bring the mixture to a boil, then reduce the heat to low and simmer for about 30-40 minutes, or until the lentils and vegetables are tender.

- Season with salt and pepper to taste.

Cooking Time: 30-40 minutes

Total Preparation Time: Approximately 45 minutes

Portion Size: Serves 4

Nutrition Value (per serving):
Calories: Approximately 250
Protein: Approximately 15g
Carbohydrates: Approximately 45g
Fat: Approximately 1g
Fiber: Approximately 15g

<u>Black Bean Burgers with Sweet Potato Fries:</u>

Ingredients:

- 1 can black beans, drained and rinsed.

- 1/2 cup cooked quinoa

- 1/2 cup finely chopped onion.

- 1/4 cup finely chopped bell pepper.

- 1 teaspoon cumin

- 1 teaspoon chili powder

- Salt and pepper to taste

- 2 medium sweet potatoes, sliced into fries.

- 1 tablespoon olive oil

Preparation Method:

- Use a fork to mash the black beans in a big bowl.

- Stir in the cooked quinoa, chopped onion, chopped bell pepper, cumin, chili powder, salt, and pepper until well combined.

- Form the mixture into burger patties.

- Preheat the oven to 400°F (200°C). Toss the sweet potato fries with olive oil and spread them out on a baking sheet.

- Bake the sweet potato fries for about 20-25 minutes, or until golden and crispy.

- While the fries are baking, cook the black bean burgers on a skillet over medium heat for about 4-5 minutes per side, or until heated through and lightly browned.

Cooking Time: Approximately 25 minutes for fries, 10 minutes for burgers

Total Preparation Time: Approximately 45 minutes

Portion Size: Serves 4

Nutrition Value (per serving, including fries and one burger):

Calories: Approximately 350

Protein: Approximately 10g
Carbohydrates: Approximately 60g
Fat: Approximately 7g
Fiber: Approximately 12g

Tofu Scramble Breakfast Burrito:

Ingredients:

- 1 block firm tofu, crumbled.
- 1 tablespoon olive oil
- 1/2 onion, chopped.
- 1/2 bell pepper, chopped.
- 1/2 cup chopped spinach.
- 1/2 teaspoon turmeric
- Salt and pepper to taste
- 4 whole wheat tortillas
- Salsa, avocado, or other desired toppings

Preparation Method:

- In a skillet over medium heat, warm the olive oil. Add the chopped onion and bell pepper and sauté until softened.
- Add the crumbled tofu, chopped spinach, turmeric, salt, and pepper to the skillet. Cook for about 5-7 minutes, stirring occasionally, until the tofu is heated through, and the spinach is wilted.

- Warm the tortillas in the skillet or microwave.

- Divide the tofu scramble mixture among the tortillas. Add desired toppings such as salsa or avocado.

- Form the tortillas into burritos and proceed to serve.

Cooking Time: Approximately 10 minutes

Total Preparation Time: Approximately 15 minutes

Portion Size: Serves 4

Nutrition Value (per serving, including one burrito):
Calories: Approximately 250
Protein: Approximately 12g
Carbohydrates: Approximately 30g
Fat: Approximately 10g
Fiber: Approximately 5g

<u>Vegetable Frittata:</u>

Ingredients:

- 6 eggs
- 1/4 cup low-fat milk
- 1 tablespoon olive oil
- 1/2 onion, chopped.
- 1 bell pepper, chopped.
- 1 cup chopped spinach.
- Salt and pepper to taste
- 1/4 cup grated cheese (optional)

Preparation Method:

- Preheat the oven to 350°F (175°C).

- In a bowl, whisk together the eggs and low-fat milk. Season with salt and pepper.

- In a skillet that is oven safe, warm the olive oil over medium heat. Add the bell pepper and onion, cut into pieces, and cook until tender.

- Cook the spinach in the skillet once it has been chopped until it wilts.

- Over the veggies in the skillet, pour the egg mixture. Cook until the edges begin to set, a few minutes.

- Sprinkle grated cheese (if using) over the top of the frittata.

- Transfer the skillet to the preheated oven and bake for about 15-20 minutes, or until the frittata is set and golden on top.

- Slice and serve.

Cooking Time: Approximately 20 minutes

Total Preparation Time: Approximately 30 minutes

Portion Size: Serves 4

Nutrition Value (per serving):
Calories: Approximately 150
Protein: Approximately 10g
Carbohydrates: Approximately 5g
Fat: Approximately 8g
Fiber: Approximately 2g

<u>Spicy Peanut Noodles:</u>

Ingredients:

- 8 oz (225g) rice noodles

- 2 tablespoons peanut butter

- 2 tablespoons low-sodium soy sauce

- 1 tablespoon rice vinegar

- 1 tablespoon sesame oil

- 1 teaspoon sriracha sauce (adjust to taste)

- 1/2 cup thinly sliced bell peppers.

- 1/2 cup shredded carrots

- 2 green onions, chopped.

- Chopped peanuts and cilantro for garnish (optional)

Preparation Method:

- Cook the rice noodles according to package instructions. Drain and set aside.

- In a small bowl, whisk together the peanut butter, soy sauce, rice vinegar, sesame oil, and sriracha sauce until smooth.

- In a large bowl, combine the cooked noodles with the sliced bell peppers, shredded carrots, and chopped green onions.

- Pour the peanut sauce over the noodles and vegetables. Toss until everything is evenly coated.

- Serve the noodles garnished with chopped peanuts and cilantro, if desired.

Cooking Time: Approximately 10 minutes

Total Preparation Time: Approximately 20 minutes

Portion Size: Serves 4

Nutrition Value (per serving):
Calories: Approximately 300
Protein: Approximately 8g
Carbohydrates: Approximately 40g
Fat: Approximately 12g
Fiber: Approximately 4g

DRINKS AND BEVERAGES

Hydration Strategies for Gastroparesis Management

Hydration is essential for overall health and can be particularly important for individuals with gastroparesis. ***Here are some hydration strategies for managing gastroparesis effectively:***

Sip fluids throughout the day: Rather than drinking large amounts of fluids at once, aim to sip fluids slowly and steadily throughout the day. This approach can help prevent overwhelming the stomach and minimize discomfort.

Choose hydrating fluids: opt for fluids that provide hydration without adding excess sugar or caffeine, which can exacerbate gastroparesis symptoms. Good choices include water, herbal teas, diluted fruit juices, and electrolyte drinks.

Monitor electrolyte balance: Gastroparesis can sometimes lead to electrolyte imbalances, particularly if vomiting or diarrhea occurs. Keep an eye on your electrolyte levels and consider incorporating electrolyte-rich foods or beverages, such as coconut water or electrolyte replacement drinks, if needed.

Experiment with temperature: Some individuals with gastroparesis find that consuming fluids at room temperature or slightly warm can be more comfortable and easier to tolerate than very cold or very hot liquids. Try a few different temperatures to discover what suits you the best.

Use a straw: Drinking through a straw can help control the flow of fluids and make it easier to manage smaller sips, especially if you have trouble swallowing or nausea.

Consider liquid meals: If solid foods are challenging to digest, liquid meals such as smoothies, soups, and broths can provide both hydration and nutrition in an easily digestible form.

Track fluid intake: Keep track of your fluid intake throughout the day to ensure you're staying adequately hydrated. This can be especially important if you're experiencing symptoms like vomiting or diarrhea, which can increase the risk of dehydration.

Consult with a healthcare provider: If you have concerns about hydration or are experiencing persistent symptoms related to gastroparesis, it's important to discuss them with your healthcare provider. They can offer personalized advice and may recommend additional interventions or treatments to help manage your symptoms effectively.

Healthy and Comforting Drinks to Choose:

Honey-Lemon Ginger Tea

Ingredients:

- 1 cup water
- One inch of freshly peeled and grated ginger
- 1/2 lemon, juiced.
- 1 teaspoon honey (optional)

Preparation Method:

- In a saucepan, heat water over medium heat until simmering.
- Simmer for five minutes after adding the grated ginger.
- Take the tea from the stove and filter it into a mug.
- Add the honey and lemon juice, if using, and stir.

Cooking Time: 5 minutes

Total Preparation Time: 10 minutes

Portion Size: 1 cup.

Nutrition Value (approximate per serving):
Calories: 3 (without honey) / 17 (with honey)
Fat: 0g
Carbohydrates: 1g (without honey) / 4g (with honey)
Protein: 0g
Sodium: 0mg

Low-Fat Yogurt Smoothie

Ingredients:

- 1 cup low-fat yogurt (plain or with fruit puree)
- 1/2 cup low-fat milk or water
- Optional additions:
- 1/4 cup frozen banana (peeled and sliced)

- 1/4 cup chopped ripe mango.

- 1/4 teaspoon ground cinnamon

Preparation Method:

- In a blender, combine yogurt and milk or water.

- Add any optional ingredients you desire.

- Blend until smooth and creamy.

Total Preparation Time: 5 minutes

Portion Size: 1 cup.

Nutrition Value (approximate per serving, plain yogurt, and milk):
Calories: 140
Fat: 3g
Carbohydrates: 18g
Protein: 8g
Sodium: 80mg

Note: Adding fruit or other ingredients will increase the calorie and carbohydrate content.

Cucumber Mint Cooler

Ingredients:

- 1/2 cup chopped cucumber.

- 4-5 fresh mint leaves

- 1 cup water

- 1/2 lemon, juiced (optional)

Preparation Method:

- In a glass, muddle the cucumber and mint leaves with a spoon to release the flavors.

- Fill the glass with water and ice.

- Add lemon juice (optional) and stir.

Total Preparation Time: 5 minutes

Portion Size: 1 cup.

Nutrition Value (approximate per serving):
Calories: 5

Fat: 0g
Carbohydrates: 1g
Protein: 0g
Sodium: 0mg

Homemade electrolyte replenishes:

Coconut Water with a Pinch of Salt:

Ingredients:

- 1 cup unsweetened coconut water
- Pinch of Himalayan pink salt (or regular table salt)

Preparation Method:

- Pour 1 cup of unsweetened coconut water into a glass.
- Add a pinch of Himalayan pink salt (or table salt) to the coconut water.
- Stir gently to dissolve the salt.

Total Preparation Time: 2 minutes

Portion Size: 1 cup.

Nutrition Value (per serving):
Calories: 46
Carbohydrates: 11g
Sodium: 45mg (can vary depending on the type of salt used)
Potassium: 200mg

Strained Watermelon Juice with a Splash of Low-Fat Milk:

Ingredients:

- 2 cups seedless watermelon, chopped.
- 1/4 cup low-fat milk (or unsweetened almond milk)
- Optional: Pinch of lime juice

Preparation Method:

- Blend the chopped watermelon in a blender until liquefied.

- Strain the watermelon juice through a fine-mesh sieve to remove pulp.

- Add the strained watermelon juice to a glass.

- Stir in 1/4 cup of low-fat milk (or unsweetened almond milk).

- Add a pinch of lime juice for extra flavor (optional).

Total Preparation Time: 5 minutes

Portion Size: 1 cup.

Nutrition Value (per serving):
Calories: 40 (may vary depending on the type of milk used)
Carbohydrates: 10g
Protein: 1g (from milk)
Potassium: 168mg

Banana and Yogurt Electrolyte Drink:

Ingredients:

- 1 ripe banana peeled and frozen.

- 1/2 cup low-fat yogurt (plain or with low-fiber fruit puree)

- 1/4 cup water

- Pinch of Himalayan pink salt (or regular table salt)

Preparation Method:

- Place the frozen banana, low-fat yogurt, water, and pinch of salt in a blender.

- Blend until smooth and creamy.

- Enjoy immediately.

Total Preparation Time: 5 minutes

Portion Size: 1 cup.

Nutrition Value (per serving):
Calories: 180 (may vary depending on the type of yogurt used)
Carbohydrates: 30g

Protein: 8g (from yogurt)
Potassium: 422mg
Sodium: 45mg (can vary depending on the type of salt used)

Non-Alcoholic Drink Recipes for Special Occasions:

Sparkling Peach Cooler:

Ingredients:

- 1 cup strained peach juice.

- 1/2 cup low-fat ginger ale

- Ice cubes.

- Fresh mint leaves for garnish (optional)

Preparation Method:

- In a pitcher, combine strained peach juice and low-fat ginger ale.

- Stir well to mix.

- Serve over ice cubes in glasses.

- Garnish with fresh mint leaves, if desired.

- Enjoy your refreshing Sparkling Peach Cooler!

Total Preparation Time: 5 minutes

Portion Size: 1 serving (approximately 1 cup)

Nutrition Value (per serving):
Calories: 80
Carbohydrates: 20g
Sugars: 18g

| Fat: 0g |
| Protein: 0g |
| Fiber: 0g |

<u>Cranberry Spritzer:</u>

Ingredients:

- 1/2 cup strained cranberry juice.

- 1/2 cup low-fat club soda

- Ice cubes.

- Fresh cranberries or orange slices for garnish (optional)

Preparation Method:

- In a glass, combine strained cranberry juice and low-fat club soda.

- Stir gently to mix.

- Serve over ice cubes.

- Garnish with fresh cranberries or orange slices, if desired.

- Enjoy your Festive Cranberry Spritzer!

Total Preparation Time: 5 minutes

Portion Size: 1 serving (approximately 1 cup)

| **Nutrition Value (per serving):** |
| Calories: 40 |
| Carbohydrates: 10g |

Sugars: 8g	
Fat: 0g	
Protein: 0g	
Fiber: 0g	

Creamy Mango Lassi:

Ingredients:

- 1 ripe mango peeled and diced.

- 1/2 cup low-fat yogurt

- 1/4 cup low-fat milk

- 1 tablespoon honey (optional)

- Ice cubes.

- Ground cardamom for garnish (optional)

Preparation Method:

- In a blender, combine diced mango, low-fat yogurt, low-fat milk, and honey (if using).

- Blend until smooth and creamy.

- Add ice cubes and blend again until well combined.

- Pour into glasses.

- Sprinkle with ground cardamom for garnish, if desired.

- Enjoy your Creamy Mango Lassi!

Total Preparation Time: 10 minutes

Portion Size: 1 serving (approximately 1 cup)

Nutrition Value (per serving):
Calories: 120
Carbohydrates: 28g
Sugars: 25g
Fat: 1g
Protein: 4g
Fiber: 2g

Spiced Apple Cider:

Ingredients:

- 2 cups unsweetened apple juice

- 1 cinnamon stick

- 3 whole cloves

- 1/4 teaspoon ground nutmeg

- 1/4 teaspoon ground allspice

- Honey or stevia to taste (optional)

- Fresh apple slices for garnish (optional)

Preparation Method:

- In a saucepan, combine unsweetened apple juice, cinnamon stick, whole cloves, ground nutmeg, and ground allspice.

- Bring to a simmer over medium heat.

- Reduce heat to low and let simmer for 10-15 minutes to allow flavors to infuse.

- Remove and filter to get rid of the spices.

- If preferred, sweeten with honey or stevia.

- Serve hot in mugs.

- Garnish with fresh apple slices, if desired.

- Enjoy your Spiced Apple Cider!

Cooking Time: 15 minutes

Total Preparation Time: 20 minutes

Portion Size: 1 serving (approximately 1 cup)

Nutrition Value (per serving):
Calories: 100
Carbohydrates: 26g
Sugars: 22g
Fat: 0g
Protein: 0g
Fiber: 0g

Tips for Everyday Living

Grocery Shopping List and Ingredient Selection Tips:

Gastroparesis requires careful planning when it comes to grocery shopping. *Here are some tips to help you build a balanced and manageable list:*

Focus on Soft and Easily Digestible Foods: Choose low-fiber fruits and vegetables, well-cooked options, and lean protein sources. Canned fruits (without added sugar) can be a good option as they are already softened. Stock up on broth-based soups, yogurt, mashed potatoes, ripe bananas, and cooked carrots.

Prioritize Protein: Protein helps you feel full for longer and is essential for maintaining muscle mass. opt for lean protein sources like skinless chicken, fish, turkey, ground meat, eggs, and low-fat yogurt.

Limited Grains and Starches: While important for energy, grains and starches can sometimes be difficult to digest in larger quantities. Choose white bread, refined cereals, white rice, and pasta over whole-wheat options. opt for smaller portions and pair them with protein and healthy fats for better digestion.

Healthy Fats: Include limited amounts of healthy fats in your diet as they can help with satiety and nutrient absorption. opt for olive oil, canola oil, or avocado oil for cooking and include avocados in your diet for a creamy and healthy fat source.

Hydration is Key: Gastroparesis can sometimes lead to dehydration. Choose hydrating liquids like water, coconut water (unsweetened), strained fruit and vegetable juices, and low-fat milk.

Read Food Labels: Pay close attention to fiber content. Look for options labeled "low fiber" or "strained." Avoid processed foods with high sugar and sodium content.

Shop in Season: Seasonal produce is often fresher and more flavorful. opt for ripe fruits and vegetables that are naturally soft and easier to digest.

Small and Frequent Meals: Plan for smaller, more frequent meals throughout the day to reduce strain on your digestive system.

Plan: Make a list before you go shopping to avoid impulse purchases that might not be gastroparesis friendly. Consider online grocery shopping or delivery services to save time and energy.

Maintaining a Balanced Diet and Nutritional Intake:

Eating a balanced diet with adequate nutrition is crucial for managing gastroparesis. Here are some pointers to help you do this:

Variety is key Include a variety of foods from different food groups in your diet to ensure you're getting all the essential nutrients.

Portion Control: Focus on smaller, more frequent meals throughout the day. This helps with digestion and prevents feeling overly full.

Blending and Pureeing: Consider blending or pureeing some of your foods to make them easier to digest. This can be done with fruits, vegetables, cooked meats, and even some cooked starches like potatoes.

Fluids with Meals: Avoid drinking large amounts of fluids directly before or during meals as this can dilute digestive juices. opt for small sips throughout the day or wait at least 30 minutes after eating to drink.

Chew Thoroughly: Take your time and chew your food thoroughly before swallowing. This helps break down food particles for easier digestion.

Listen to Your Body: Observe how various foods affect your body's response. If you experience discomfort after eating something, avoid it in the future.

Work with a Dietitian: Consulting a registered dietitian can be invaluable for creating a personalized meal plan that addresses your specific needs and preferences. They can also offer guidance on portion sizes, blending techniques, and dietary supplements if needed.

Additional Tips:

Cooking Methods: opt for cooking methods that make food softer and easier to digest, such as steaming, poaching, baking, and simmering.

Ginger: Ginger is known for its digestive properties. Consider incorporating ginger into your diet in small amounts, such as adding it to stir-fries or teas.

Pro biotic: Pro biotics may help improve gut health and digestion. Talk to your doctor about whether pro biotic supplements might be beneficial for you.

Remember, managing gastroparesis requires ongoing adjustments and learning what works best for you. Don't get discouraged if you experience setbacks. By following these tips and working with your healthcare team, you can maintain a healthy and balanced diet that supports your well-being.

Conclusion

Living with gastroparesis can be a daily challenge, but it doesn't have to define your life.

Throughout this book, we've explored the condition, its management strategies, and delicious recipes you can enjoy. Remember, you're not alone on this journey. There's a supportive community of people navigating similar experiences, and a wealth of resources available to you. As you move forward, embrace the power of small wins. Celebrate each symptom-free day, each delicious and nourishing meal you consume. Don't be afraid to experiment with flavors and textures within your dietary guidelines. Remember, a balanced diet doesn't have to be bland. This book has equipped you with the knowledge and tools to navigate gastroparesis with confidence. Embrace a positive outlook, prioritize self-care, and don't hesitate to seek support from your healthcare team and loved ones. With a proactive approach and a touch of creativity, you can find joy, energy, and a sense of control in managing your gastroparesis. Remember, a healthy and fulfilling life is possible. Now, go out there and create delicious memories, one gastroparesis-friendly bite at a time!

Now let's move to the bonus section.

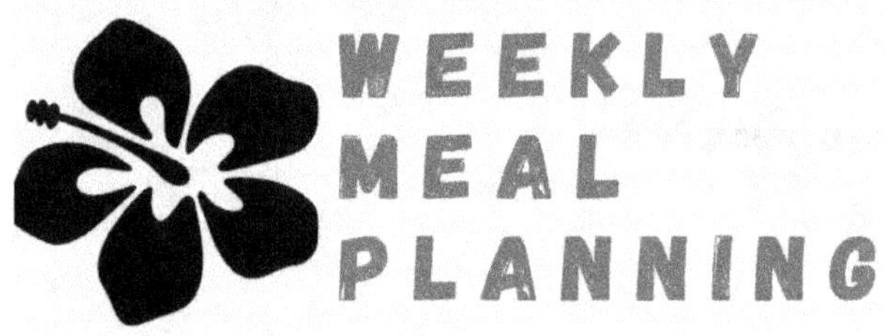

Month:

Week:

(1) (2) (3) (4)

Sunday

Breakfast: __________

Calories	Protein	Sugar	Carbs

Lunch: __________

Calories	Protein	Sugar	Carbs

Dinner: __________

Calories	Protein	Sugar	Carbs

Monday

Breakfast: __________

Calories	Protein	Sugar	Carbs

Lunch: __________

Calories	Protein	Sugar	Carbs

Dinner: __________

Calories	Protein	Sugar	Carbs

Tuesday

Breakfast: __________

Calories	Protein	Sugar	Carbs

Lunch: __________

Calories	Protein	Sugar	Carbs

Dinner: __________

Calories	Protein	Sugar	Carbs

Wednesday

Breakfast: __________

Calories	Protein	Sugar	Carbs

Lunch: __________

Calories	Protein	Sugar	Carbs

Dinner: __________

Calories	Protein	Sugar	Carbs

Thursday

Breakfast: __________

Calories	Protein	Carbs

Lunch: __________

Calories	Protein	Sugar	Carbs

Dinner: __________

Calories	Protein	Sugar	Carbs

Friday

Breakfast: __________

Calories	Protein	Sugar	Carbs

Lunch: __________

Calories	Protein	Sugar	Carbs

Dinner: __________

Calories	Protein	Sugar	Carbs

Saturday

Breakfast: __________

Calories	Protein	Sugar	Carbs

Lunch: __________

Calories	Protein	Sugar	Carbs

Dinner: __________

Calories	Protein	Sugar	Carbs

Shopping List:

____

____

____

____

____

____

____

____

____

____

____

____

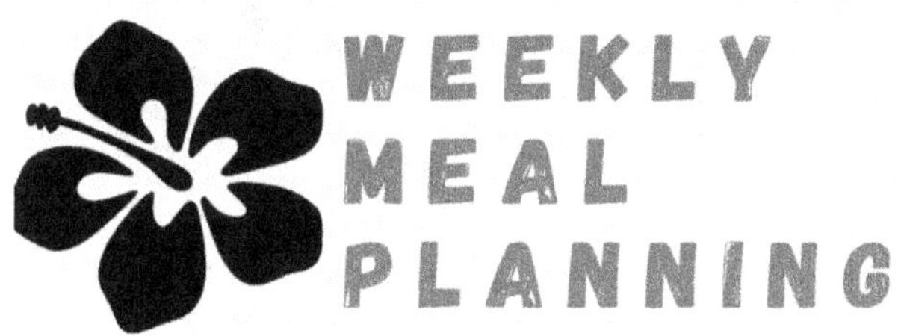

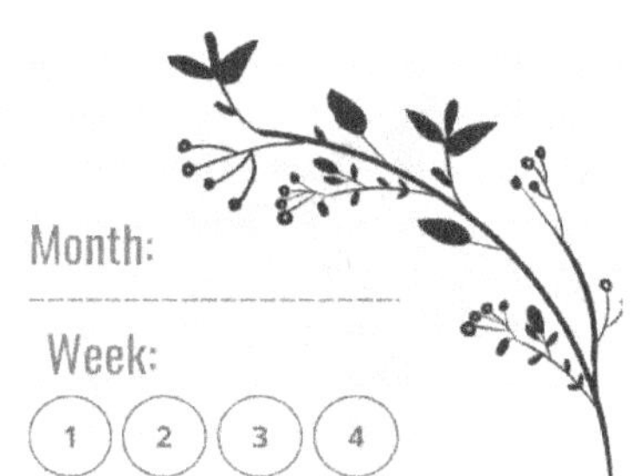

Month: ___________

Week: ① ② ③ ④

Sunday

Breakfast: _______________

Calories	Protein	Sugar	Carbs

Lunch: _______________

Calories	Protein	Sugar	Carbs

Dinner: _______________

Calories	Protein	Sugar	Carbs

Monday

Breakfast: _______________

Calories	Protein	Sugar	Carbs

Lunch: _______________

Calories	Protein	Sugar	Carbs

Dinner: _______________

Calories	Protein	Sugar	Carbs

Tuesday

Breakfast: _______________

Calories	Protein	Sugar	Carbs

Lunch: _______________

Calories	Protein	Sugar	Carbs

Dinner: _______________

Calories	Protein	Sugar	Carbs

Wednesday

Breakfast: _______________

Calories	Protein	Sugar	Carbs

Lunch: _______________

Calories	Protein	Sugar	Carbs

Dinner: _______________

Calories	Protein	Sugar	Carbs

Thursday

Breakfast: _______________

Calories	Protein	Carbs

Lunch: _______________

Calories	Protein	Sugar	Carbs

Dinner: _______________

Calories	Protein	Sugar	Carbs

Friday

Breakfast: _______________

Calories	Protein	Sugar	Carbs

Lunch: _______________

Calories	Protein	Sugar	Carbs

Dinner: _______________

Calories	Protein	Sugar	Carbs

Saturday

Breakfast: _______________

Calories	Protein	Sugar	Carbs

Lunch: _______________

Calories	Protein	Sugar	Carbs

Dinner: _______________

Calories	Protein	Sugar	Carbs

Shopping List:

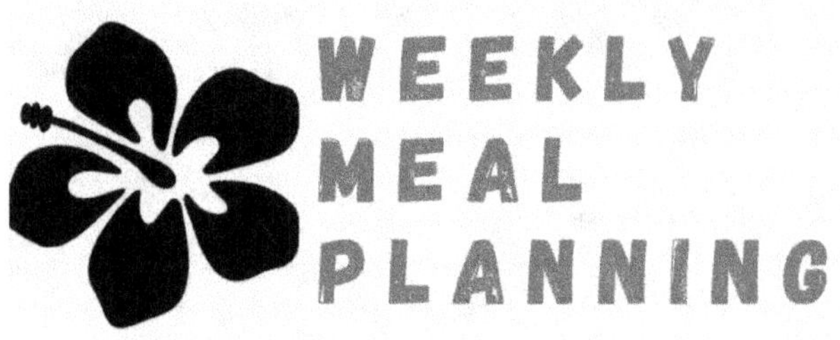

WEEKLY MEAL PLANNING

Month:

Week: 1 2 3 4

Sunday

Breakfast:

Calories	Protein	Sugar	Carbs

Lunch:

Calories	Protein	Sugar	Carbs

Dinner:

Calories	Protein	Sugar	Carbs

Monday

Breakfast:

Calories	Protein	Sugar	Carbs

Lunch:

Calories	Protein	Sugar	Carbs

Dinner:

Calories	Protein	Sugar	Carbs

Tuesday

Breakfast:

Calories	Protein	Sugar	Carbs

Lunch:

Calories	Protein	Sugar	Carbs

Dinner:

Calories	Protein	Sugar	Carbs

Wednesday

Breakfast:

Calories	Protein	Sugar	Carbs

Lunch:

Calories	Protein	Sugar	Carbs

Dinner:

Calories	Protein	Sugar	Carbs

Thursday

Breakfast:

Calories	Protein	Carbs

Lunch:

Calories	Protein	Sugar	Carbs

Dinner:

Calories	Protein	Sugar	Carbs

Friday

Breakfast:

Calories	Protein	Sugar	Carbs

Lunch:

Calories	Protein	Sugar	Carbs

Dinner:

Calories	Protein	Sugar	Carbs

Saturday

Breakfast:

Calories	Protein	Sugar	Carbs

Lunch:

Calories	Protein	Sugar	Carbs

Dinner:

Calories	Protein	Sugar	Carbs

Shopping List:

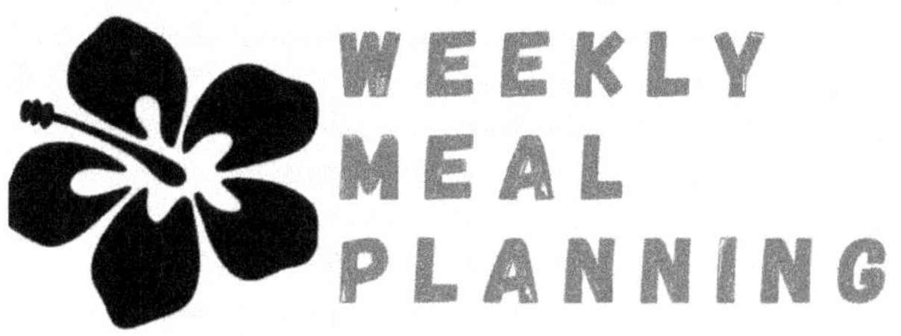
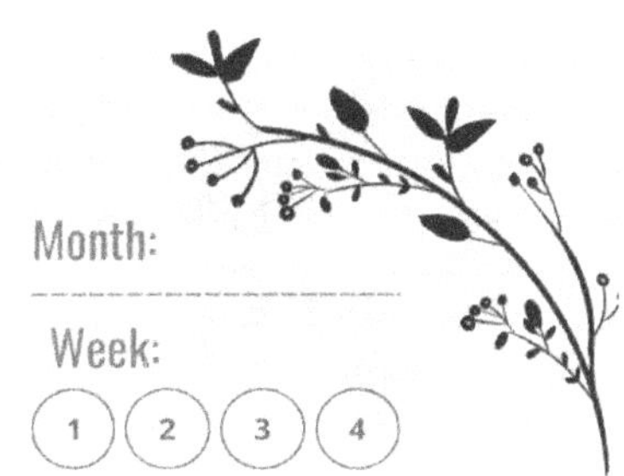

WEEKLY MEAL PLANNING

Month: _______

Week:

(1) (2) (3) (4)

Sunday

Breakfast: _______

Calories	Protein	Sugar	Carbs

Lunch: _______

Calories	Protein	Sugar	Carbs

Dinner: _______

Calories	Protein	Sugar	Carbs

Monday

Breakfast: _______

Calories	Protein	Sugar	Carbs

Lunch: _______

Calories	Protein	Sugar	Carbs

Dinner: _______

Calories	Protein	Sugar	Carbs

Tuesday

Breakfast: _______

Calories	Protein	Sugar	Carbs

Lunch: _______

Calories	Protein	Sugar	Carbs

Dinner: _______

Calories	Protein	Sugar	Carbs

Wednesday

Breakfast: _______

Calories	Protein	Sugar	Carbs

Lunch: _______

Calories	Protein	Sugar	Carbs

Dinner: _______

Calories	Protein	Sugar	Carbs

Thursday

Breakfast: _______

Calories	Protein	Carbs

Lunch: _______

Calories	Protein	Sugar	Carbs

Dinner: _______

Calories	Protein	Sugar	Carbs

Friday

Breakfast: _______

Calories	Protein	Sugar	Carbs

Lunch: _______

Calories	Protein	Sugar	Carbs

Dinner: _______

Calories	Protein	Sugar	Carbs

Saturday

Breakfast: _______

Calories	Protein	Sugar	Carbs

Lunch: _______

Calories	Protein	Sugar	Carbs

Dinner: _______

Calories	Protein	Sugar	Carbs

Shopping List:

____

____

____

____

____

____

____

____

____

____

____

____

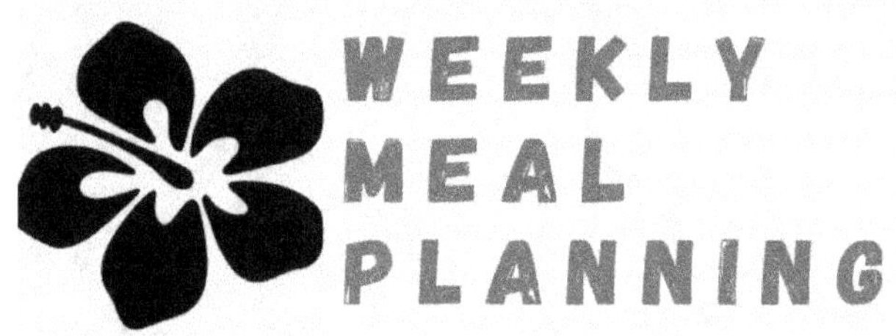

WEEKLY MEAL PLANNING

Month:

Week:

(1) (2) (3) (4)

Sunday

Breakfast:

Calories	Protein	Sugar	Carbs

Lunch:

Calories	Protein	Sugar	Carbs

Dinner:

Calories	Protein	Sugar	Carbs

Monday

Breakfast:

Calories	Protein	Sugar	Carbs

Lunch:

Calories	Protein	Sugar	Carbs

Dinner:

Calories	Protein	Sugar	Carbs

Tuesday

Breakfast:

Calories	Protein	Sugar	Carbs

Lunch:

Calories	Protein	Sugar	Carbs

Dinner:

Calories	Protein	Sugar	Carbs

Wednesday

Breakfast:

Calories	Protein	Sugar	Carbs

Lunch:

Calories	Protein	Sugar	Carbs

Dinner:

Calories	Protein	Sugar	Carbs

Thursday

Breakfast:

Calories	Protein	Carbs

Lunch:

Calories	Protein	Sugar	Carbs

Dinner:

Calories	Protein	Sugar	Carbs

Friday

Breakfast:

Calories	Protein	Sugar	Carbs

Lunch:

Calories	Protein	Sugar	Carbs

Dinner:

Calories	Protein	Sugar	Carbs

Saturday

Breakfast:

Calories	Protein	Sugar	Carbs

Lunch:

Calories	Protein	Sugar	Carbs

Dinner:

Calories	Protein	Sugar	Carbs

Shopping List:

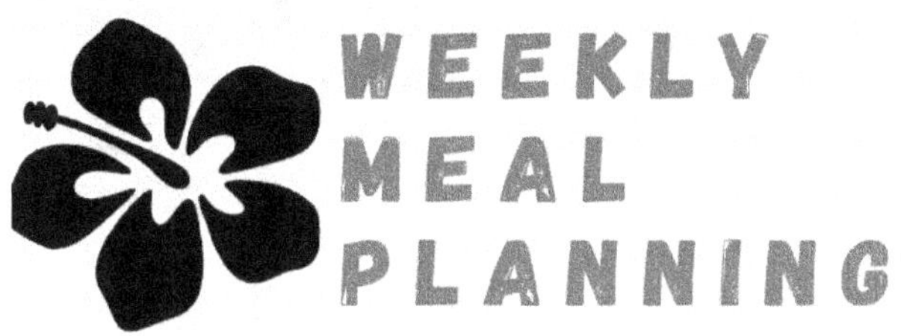

WEEKLY MEAL PLANNING

Month:

Week:
(1) (2) (3) (4)

Sunday

Breakfast:

Calories	Protein	Sugar	Carbs

Lunch:

Calories	Protein	Sugar	Carbs

Dinner:

Calories	Protein	Sugar	Carbs

Monday

Breakfast:

Calories	Protein	Sugar	Carbs

Lunch:

Calories	Protein	Sugar	Carbs

Dinner:

Calories	Protein	Sugar	Carbs

Tuesday

Breakfast:

Calories	Protein	Sugar	Carbs

Lunch:

Calories	Protein	Sugar	Carbs

Dinner:

Calories	Protein	Sugar	Carbs

Wednesday

Breakfast:

Calories	Protein	Sugar	Carbs

Lunch:

Calories	Protein	Sugar	Carbs

Dinner:

Calories	Protein	Sugar	Carbs

Thursday

Breakfast:

Calories	Protein	Carbs

Lunch:

Calories	Protein	Sugar	Carbs

Dinner:

Calories	Protein	Sugar	Carbs

Friday

Breakfast:

Calories	Protein	Sugar	Carbs

Lunch:

Calories	Protein	Sugar	Carbs

Dinner:

Calories	Protein	Sugar	Carbs

Saturday

Breakfast:

Calories	Protein	Sugar	Carbs

Lunch:

Calories	Protein	Sugar	Carbs

Dinner:

Calories	Protein	Sugar	Carbs

Shopping List:

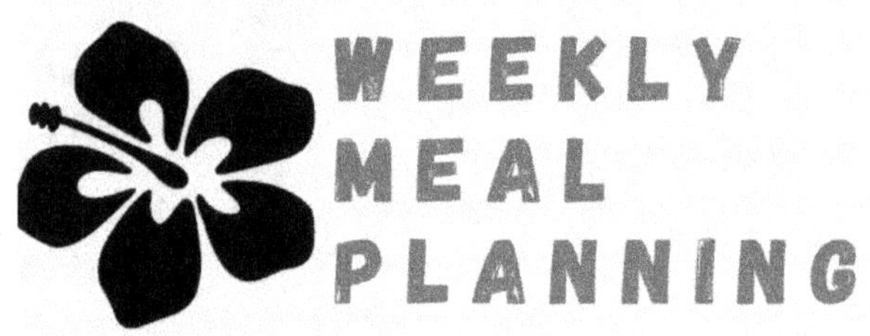

WEEKLY MEAL PLANNING

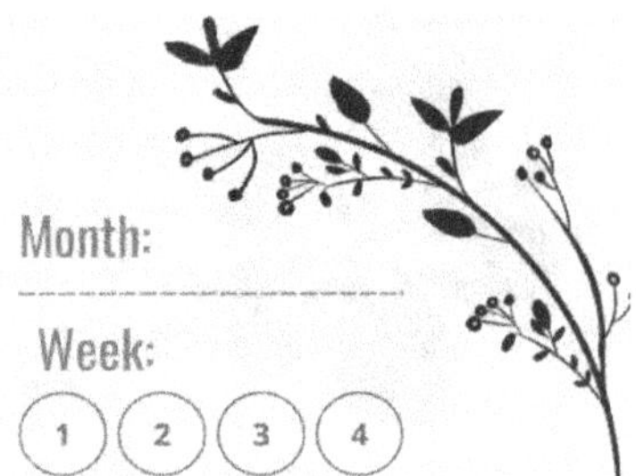

Month:

Week:
(1) (2) (3) (4)

Sunday

Breakfast:

Calories	Protein	Sugar	Carbs

Lunch:

Calories	Protein	Sugar	Carbs

Dinner:

Calories	Protein	Sugar	Carbs

Monday

Breakfast:

Calories	Protein	Sugar	Carbs

Lunch:

Calories	Protein	Sugar	Carbs

Dinner:

Calories	Protein	Sugar	Carbs

Tuesday

Breakfast:

Calories	Protein	Sugar	Carbs

Lunch:

Calories	Protein	Sugar	Carbs

Dinner:

Calories	Protein	Sugar	Carbs

Wednesday

Breakfast:

Calories	Protein	Sugar	Carbs

Lunch:

Calories	Protein	Sugar	Carbs

Dinner:

Calories	Protein	Sugar	Carbs

Thursday

Breakfast:

Calories	Protein	Carbs

Lunch:

Calories	Protein	Sugar	Carbs

Dinner:

Calories	Protein	Sugar	Carbs

Friday

Breakfast:

Calories	Protein	Sugar	Carbs

Lunch:

Calories	Protein	Sugar	Carbs

Dinner:

Calories	Protein	Sugar	Carbs

Saturday

Breakfast:

Calories	Protein	Sugar	Carbs

Lunch:

Calories	Protein	Sugar	Carbs

Dinner:

Calories	Protein	Sugar	Carbs

Shopping List:

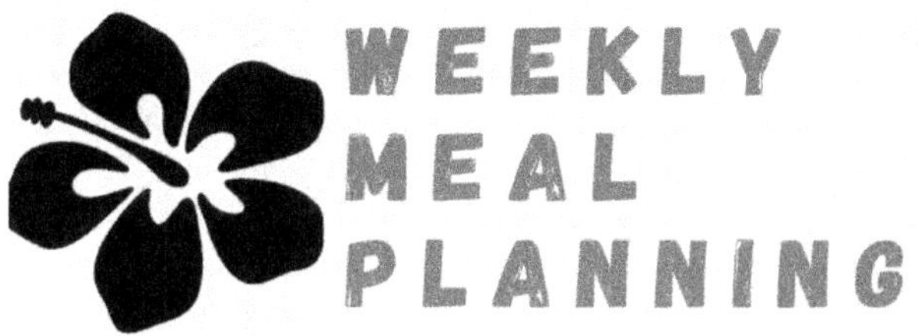

WEEKLY MEAL PLANNING

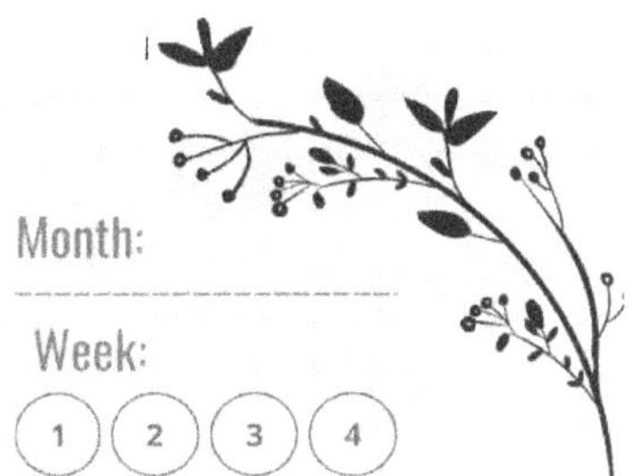

Month: ____________

Week:
(1) (2) (3) (4)

Sunday

Breakfast: ____________

Calories	Protein	Sugar	Carbs

Lunch: ____________

Calories	Protein	Sugar	Carbs

Dinner: ____________

Calories	Protein	Sugar	Carbs

Monday

Breakfast: ____________

Calories	Protein	Sugar	Carbs

Lunch: ____________

Calories	Protein	Sugar	Carbs

Dinner: ____________

Calories	Protein	Sugar	Carbs

Tuesday

Breakfast: ____________

Calories	Protein	Sugar	Carbs

Lunch: ____________

Calories	Protein	Sugar	Carbs

Dinner: ____________

Calories	Protein	Sugar	Carbs

Wednesday

Breakfast: ____________

Calories	Protein	Sugar	Carbs

Lunch: ____________

Calories	Protein	Sugar	Carbs

Dinner: ____________

Calories	Protein	Sugar	Carbs

Thursday

Breakfast: ____________

Calories	Protein		Carbs

Lunch: ____________

Calories	Protein	Sugar	Carbs

Dinner: ____________

Calories	Protein	Sugar	Carbs

Friday

Breakfast: ____________

Calories	Protein	Sugar	Carbs

Lunch: ____________

Calories	Protein	Sugar	Carbs

Dinner: ____________

Calories	Protein	Sugar	Carbs

Saturday

Breakfast: ____________

Calories	Protein	Sugar	Carbs

Lunch: ____________

Calories	Protein	Sugar	Carbs

Dinner: ____________

Calories	Protein	Sugar	Carbs

Shopping List:

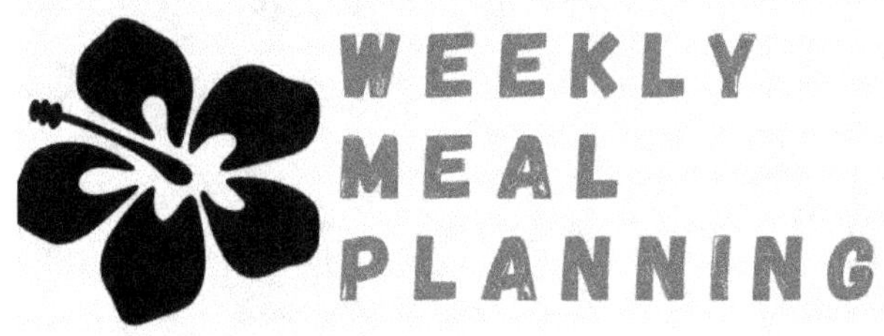

Month:

Week:

(1) (2) (3) (4)

Sunday

Breakfast:

Calories	Protein	Sugar	Carbs

Lunch:

Calories	Protein	Sugar	Carbs

Dinner:

Calories	Protein	Sugar	Carbs

Monday

Breakfast:

Calories	Protein	Sugar	Carbs

Lunch:

Calories	Protein	Sugar	Carbs

Dinner:

Calories	Protein	Sugar	Carbs

Tuesday

Breakfast:

Calories	Protein	Sugar	Carbs

Lunch:

Calories	Protein	Sugar	Carbs

Dinner:

Calories	Protein	Sugar	Carbs

Wednesday

Breakfast:

Calories	Protein	Sugar	Carbs

Lunch:

Calories	Protein	Sugar	Carbs

Dinner:

Calories	Protein	Sugar	Carbs

Thursday

Breakfast:

Calories	Protein	Carbs

Lunch:

Calories	Protein	Sugar	Carbs

Dinner:

Calories	Protein	Sugar	Carbs

Friday

Breakfast:

Calories	Protein	Sugar	Carbs

Lunch:

Calories	Protein	Sugar	Carbs

Dinner:

Calories	Protein	Sugar	Carbs

Saturday

Breakfast:

Calories	Protein	Sugar	Carbs

Lunch:

Calories	Protein	Sugar	Carbs

Dinner:

Calories	Protein	Sugar	Carbs

Shopping List:

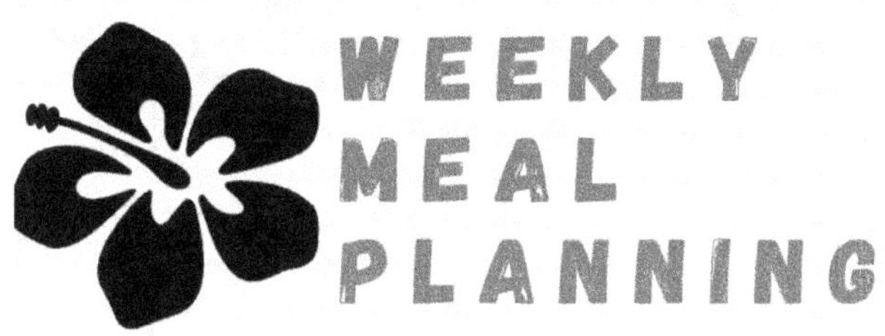

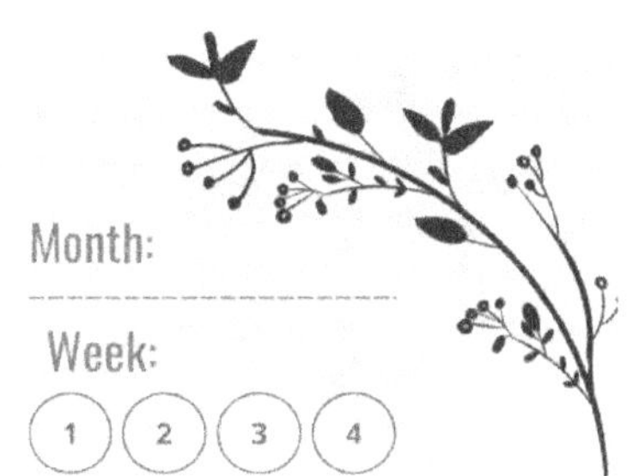

Month:

Week:

(1) (2) (3) (4)

Sunday

Breakfast:

Calories	Protein	Sugar	Carbs

Lunch:

Calories	Protein	Sugar	Carbs

Dinner:

Calories	Protein	Sugar	Carbs

Monday

Breakfast:

Calories	Protein	Sugar	Carbs

Lunch:

Calories	Protein	Sugar	Carbs

Dinner:

Calories	Protein	Sugar	Carbs

Tuesday

Breakfast:

Calories	Protein	Sugar	Carbs

Lunch:

Calories	Protein	Sugar	Carbs

Dinner:

Calories	Protein	Sugar	Carbs

Wednesday

Breakfast:

Calories	Protein	Sugar	Carbs

Lunch:

Calories	Protein	Sugar	Carbs

Dinner:

Calories	Protein	Sugar	Carbs

Thursday

Breakfast:

Calories	Protein	Carbs

Lunch:

Calories	Protein	Sugar	Carbs

Dinner:

Calories	Protein	Sugar	Carbs

Friday

Breakfast:

Calories	Protein	Sugar	Carbs

Lunch:

Calories	Protein	Sugar	Carbs

Dinner:

Calories	Protein	Sugar	Carbs

Saturday

Breakfast:

Calories	Protein	Sugar	Carbs

Lunch:

Calories	Protein	Sugar	Carbs

Dinner:

Calories	Protein	Sugar	Carbs

Shopping List:

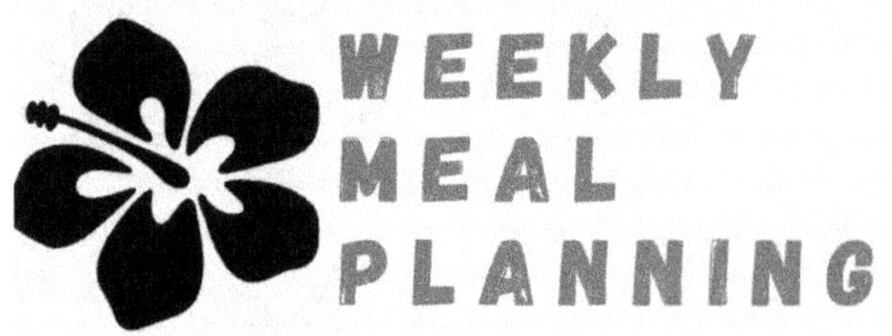

WEEKLY MEAL PLANNING

Month: __________

Week: __________

(1) (2) (3) (4)

Sunday

Breakfast: __________

Calories	Protein	Sugar	Carbs

Lunch: __________

Calories	Protein	Sugar	Carbs

Dinner: __________

Calories	Protein	Sugar	Carbs

Monday

Breakfast: __________

Calories	Protein	Sugar	Carbs

Lunch: __________

Calories	Protein	Sugar	Carbs

Dinner: __________

Calories	Protein	Sugar	Carbs

Tuesday

Breakfast: __________

Calories	Protein	Sugar	Carbs

Lunch: __________

Calories	Protein	Sugar	Carbs

Dinner: __________

Calories	Protein	Sugar	Carbs

Wednesday

Breakfast: __________

Calories	Protein	Sugar	Carbs

Lunch: __________

Calories	Protein	Sugar	Carbs

Dinner: __________

Calories	Protein	Sugar	Carbs

Thursday

Breakfast: __________

Calories	Protein	Sugar	Carbs

Lunch: __________

Calories	Protein	Sugar	Carbs

Dinner: __________

Calories	Protein	Sugar	Carbs

Friday

Breakfast: __________

Calories	Protein	Sugar	Carbs

Lunch: __________

Calories	Protein	Sugar	Carbs

Dinner: __________

Calories	Protein	Sugar	Carbs

Saturday

Breakfast: __________

Calories	Protein	Sugar	Carbs

Lunch: __________

Calories	Protein	Sugar	Carbs

Dinner: __________

Calories	Protein	Sugar	Carbs

Shopping List:

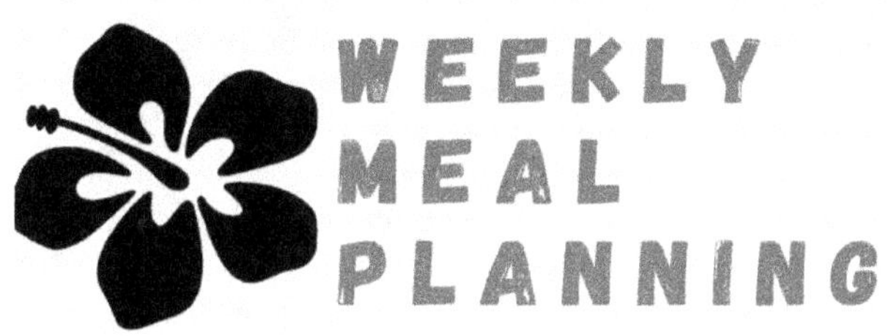

WEEKLY MEAL PLANNING

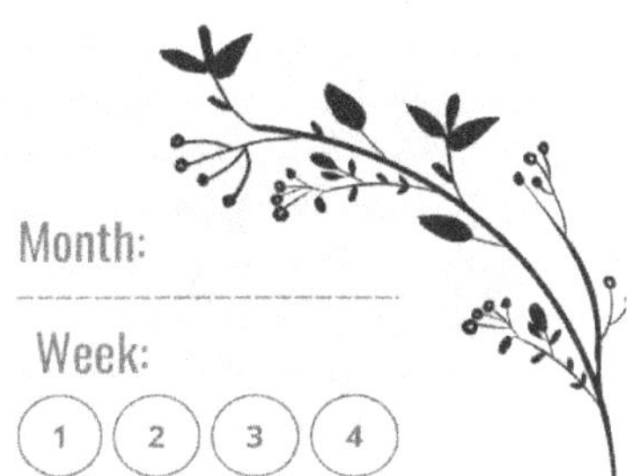

Month: _______

Week:
(1) (2) (3) (4)

Sunday

Breakfast: _______

Calories	Protein	Sugar	Carbs

Lunch: _______

Calories	Protein	Sugar	Carbs

Dinner: _______

Calories	Protein	Sugar	Carbs

Monday

Breakfast: _______

Calories	Protein	Sugar	Carbs

Lunch: _______

Calories	Protein	Sugar	Carbs

Dinner: _______

Calories	Protein	Sugar	Carbs

Tuesday

Breakfast: _______

Calories	Protein	Sugar	Carbs

Lunch: _______

Calories	Protein	Sugar	Carbs

Dinner: _______

Calories	Protein	Sugar	Carbs

Wednesday

Breakfast: _______

Calories	Protein	Sugar	Carbs

Lunch: _______

Calories	Protein	Sugar	Carbs

Dinner: _______

Calories	Protein	Sugar	Carbs

Thursday

Breakfast: _______

Calories	Protein	Carbs

Lunch: _______

Calories	Protein	Sugar	Carbs

Dinner: _______

Calories	Protein	Sugar	Carbs

Friday

Breakfast: _______

Calories	Protein	Sugar	Carbs

Lunch: _______

Calories	Protein	Sugar	Carbs

Dinner: _______

Calories	Protein	Sugar	Carbs

Saturday

Breakfast: _______

Calories	Protein	Sugar	Carbs

Lunch: _______

Calories	Protein	Sugar	Carbs

Dinner: _______

Calories	Protein	Sugar	Carbs

Shopping List:

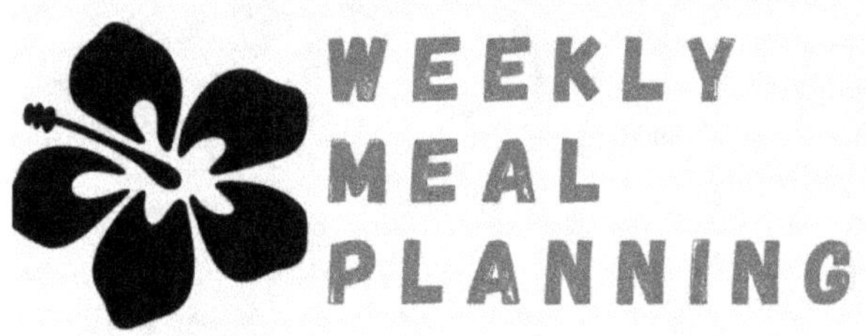

WEEKLY MEAL PLANNING

Month: _______

Week:

(1) (2) (3) (4)

Sunday

Breakfast: _______

Calories	Protein	Sugar	Carbs

Lunch: _______

Calories	Protein	Sugar	Carbs

Dinner: _______

Calories	Protein	Sugar	Carbs

Monday

Breakfast: _______

Calories	Protein	Sugar	Carbs

Lunch: _______

Calories	Protein	Sugar	Carbs

Dinner: _______

Calories	Protein	Sugar	Carbs

Tuesday

Breakfast: _______

Calories	Protein	Sugar	Carbs

Lunch: _______

Calories	Protein	Sugar	Carbs

Dinner: _______

Calories	Protein	Sugar	Carbs

Wednesday

Breakfast: _______

Calories	Protein	Sugar	Carbs

Lunch: _______

Calories	Protein	Sugar	Carbs

Dinner: _______

Calories	Protein	Sugar	Carbs

Thursday

Breakfast: _______

Calories	Protein	Carbs

Lunch: _______

Calories	Protein	Sugar	Carbs

Dinner: _______

Calories	Protein	Sugar	Carbs

Friday

Breakfast: _______

Calories	Protein	Sugar	Carbs

Lunch: _______

Calories	Protein	Sugar	Carbs

Dinner: _______

Calories	Protein	Sugar	Carbs

Saturday

Breakfast: _______

Calories	Protein	Sugar	Carbs

Lunch: _______

Calories	Protein	Sugar	Carbs

Dinner: _______

Calories	Protein	Sugar	Carbs

Shopping List:

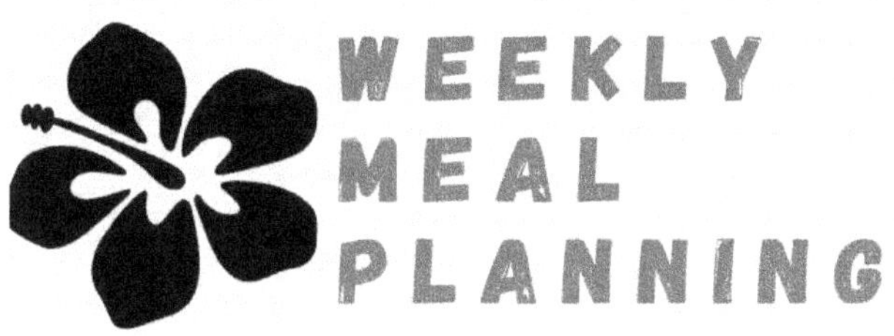

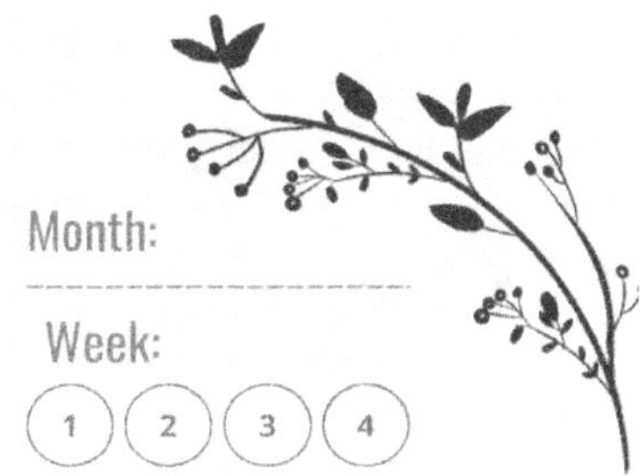

Month:

Week:

1 2 3 4

Sunday

Breakfast:

Calories	Protein	Sugar	Carbs

Lunch:

Calories	Protein	Sugar	Carbs

Dinner:

Calories	Protein	Sugar	Carbs

Monday

Breakfast:

Calories	Protein	Sugar	Carbs

Lunch:

Calories	Protein	Sugar	Carbs

Dinner:

Calories	Protein	Sugar	Carbs

Tuesday

Breakfast:

Calories	Protein	Sugar	Carbs

Lunch:

Calories	Protein	Sugar	Carbs

Dinner:

Calories	Protein	Sugar	Carbs

Wednesday

Breakfast:

Calories	Protein	Sugar	Carbs

Lunch:

Calories	Protein	Sugar	Carbs

Dinner:

Calories	Protein	Sugar	Carbs

Thursday

Breakfast:

Calories	Protein	Carbs

Lunch:

Calories	Protein	Sugar	Carbs

Dinner:

Calories	Protein	Sugar	Carbs

Friday

Breakfast:

Calories	Protein	Sugar	Carbs

Lunch:

Calories	Protein	Sugar	Carbs

Dinner:

Calories	Protein	Sugar	Carbs

Saturday

Breakfast:

Calories	Protein	Sugar	Carbs

Lunch:

Calories	Protein	Sugar	Carbs

Dinner:

Calories	Protein	Sugar	Carbs

Shopping List:

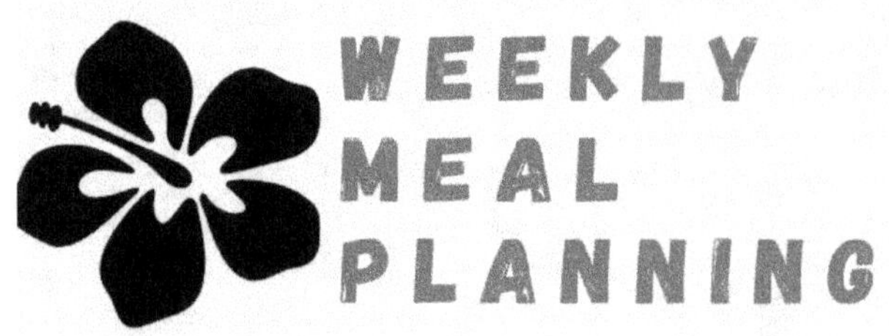

WEEKLY MEAL PLANNING

Month: ______

Week: (1) (2) (3) (4)

Sunday

Breakfast: ______

Calories	Protein	Sugar	Carbs

Lunch: ______

Calories	Protein	Sugar	Carbs

Dinner: ______

Calories	Protein	Sugar	Carbs

Monday

Breakfast: ______

Calories	Protein	Sugar	Carbs

Lunch: ______

Calories	Protein	Sugar	Carbs

Dinner: ______

Calories	Protein	Sugar	Carbs

Tuesday

Breakfast: ______

Calories	Protein	Sugar	Carbs

Lunch: ______

Calories	Protein	Sugar	Carbs

Dinner: ______

Calories	Protein	Sugar	Carbs

Wednesday

Breakfast: ______

Calories	Protein	Sugar	Carbs

Lunch: ______

Calories	Protein	Sugar	Carbs

Dinner: ______

Calories	Protein	Sugar	Carbs

Thursday

Breakfast: ______

Calories	Protein		Carbs

Lunch: ______

Calories	Protein	Sugar	Carbs

Dinner: ______

Calories	Protein	Sugar	Carbs

Friday

Breakfast: ______

Calories	Protein	Sugar	Carbs

Lunch: ______

Calories	Protein	Sugar	Carbs

Dinner: ______

Calories	Protein	Sugar	Carbs

Saturday

Breakfast: ______

Calories	Protein	Sugar	Carbs

Lunch: ______

Calories	Protein	Sugar	Carbs

Dinner: ______

Calories	Protein	Sugar	Carbs

Shopping List:

____
____
____
____
____
____
____
____
____
____

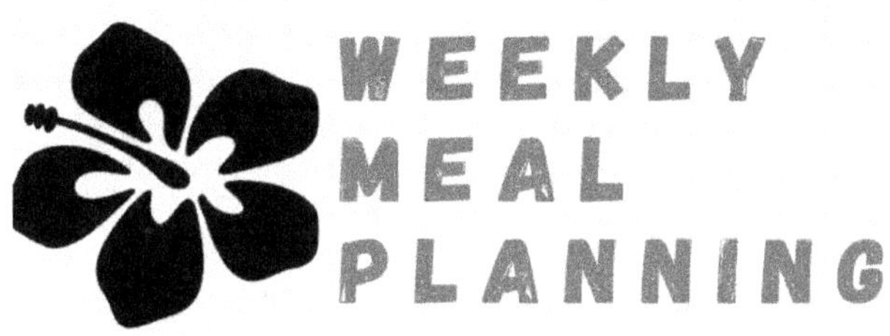

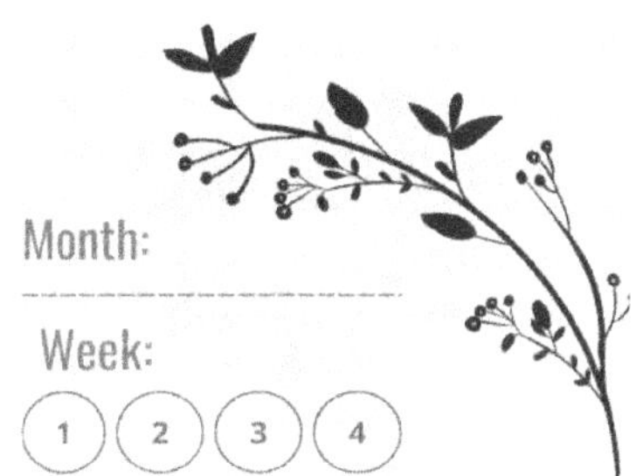

Month:

Week:
(1) (2) (3) (4)

Sunday

Breakfast:

Calories	Protein	Sugar	Carbs

Lunch:

Calories	Protein	Sugar	Carbs

Dinner:

Calories	Protein	Sugar	Carbs

Monday

Breakfast:

Calories	Protein	Sugar	Carbs

Lunch:

Calories	Protein	Sugar	Carbs

Dinner:

Calories	Protein	Sugar	Carbs

Tuesday

Breakfast:

Calories	Protein	Sugar	Carbs

Lunch:

Calories	Protein	Sugar	Carbs

Dinner:

Calories	Protein	Sugar	Carbs

Wednesday

Breakfast:

Calories	Protein	Sugar	Carbs

Lunch:

Calories	Protein	Sugar	Carbs

Dinner:

Calories	Protein	Sugar	Carbs

Thursday

Breakfast:

Calories	Protein	Carbs

Lunch:

Calories	Protein	Sugar	Carbs

Dinner:

Calories	Protein	Sugar	Carbs

Friday

Breakfast:

Calories	Protein	Sugar	Carbs

Lunch:

Calories	Protein	Sugar	Carbs

Dinner:

Calories	Protein	Sugar	Carbs

Saturday

Breakfast:

Calories	Protein	Sugar	Carbs

Lunch:

Calories	Protein	Sugar	Carbs

Dinner:

Calories	Protein	Sugar	Carbs

Shopping List:

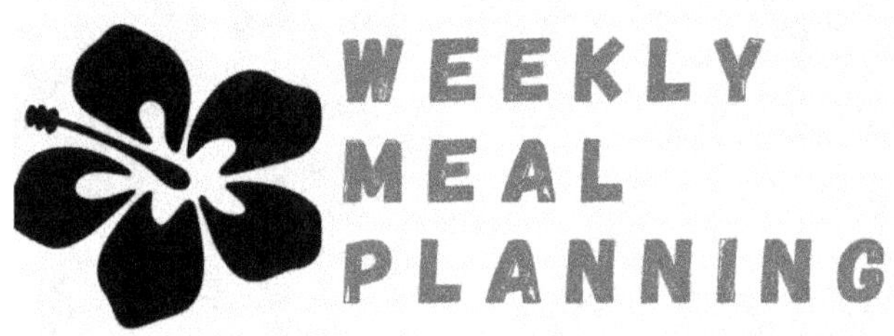

WEEKLY MEAL PLANNING

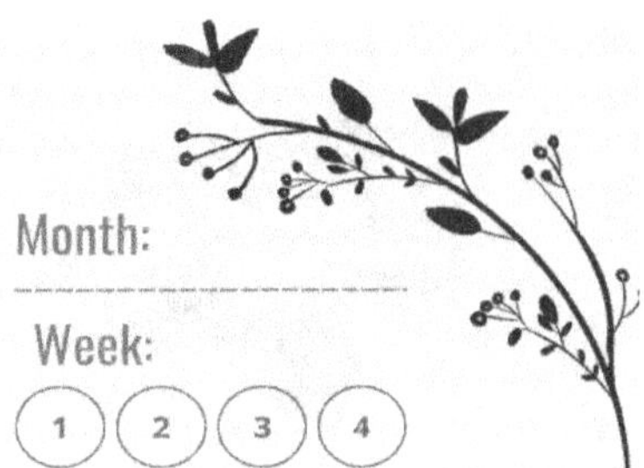

Month:

Week:

(1) (2) (3) (4)

Sunday

Breakfast:

Calories	Protein	Sugar	Carbs

Lunch:

Calories	Protein	Sugar	Carbs

Dinner:

Calories	Protein	Sugar	Carbs

Monday

Breakfast:

Calories	Protein	Sugar	Carbs

Lunch:

Calories	Protein	Sugar	Carbs

Dinner:

Calories	Protein	Sugar	Carbs

Tuesday

Breakfast:

Calories	Protein	Sugar	Carbs

Lunch:

Calories	Protein	Sugar	Carbs

Dinner:

Calories	Protein	Sugar	Carbs

Wednesday

Breakfast:

Calories	Protein	Sugar	Carbs

Lunch:

Calories	Protein	Sugar	Carbs

Dinner:

Calories	Protein	Sugar	Carbs

Thursday

Breakfast:

Calories	Protein	Carbs

Lunch:

Calories	Protein	Sugar	Carbs

Dinner:

Calories	Protein	Sugar	Carbs

Friday

Breakfast:

Calories	Protein	Sugar	Carbs

Lunch:

Calories	Protein	Sugar	Carbs

Dinner:

Calories	Protein	Sugar	Carbs

Saturday

Breakfast:

Calories	Protein	Sugar	Carbs

Lunch:

Calories	Protein	Sugar	Carbs

Dinner:

Calories	Protein	Sugar	Carbs

Shopping List:

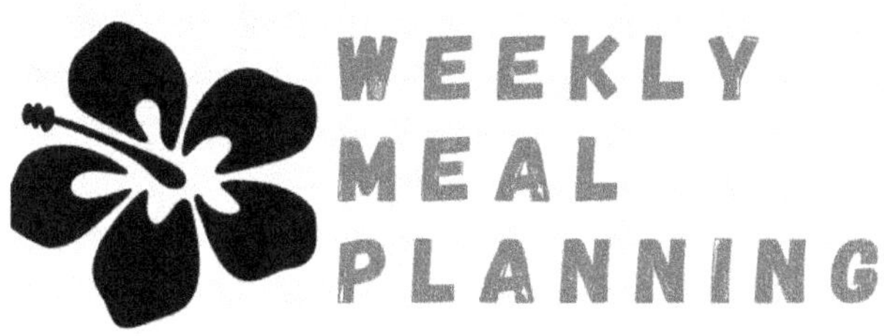

WEEKLY MEAL PLANNING

Month:

Week:
1 2 3 4

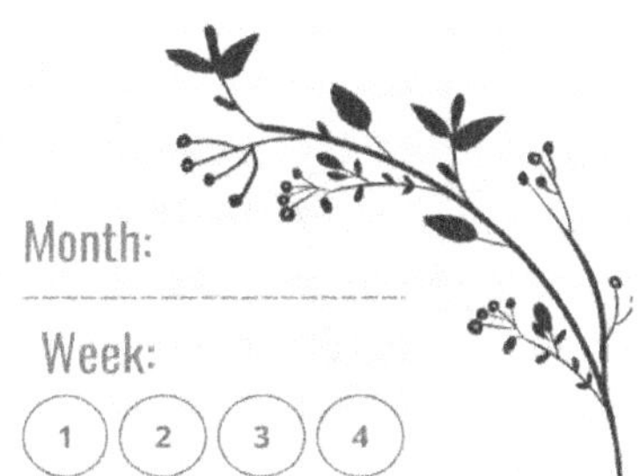

Sunday

Breakfast:

Calories	Protein	Sugar	Carbs

Lunch:

Calories	Protein	Sugar	Carbs

Dinner:

Calories	Protein	Sugar	Carbs

Monday

Breakfast:

Calories	Protein	Sugar	Carbs

Lunch:

Calories	Protein	Sugar	Carbs

Dinner:

Calories	Protein	Sugar	Carbs

Tuesday

Breakfast:

Calories	Protein	Sugar	Carbs

Lunch:

Calories	Protein	Sugar	Carbs

Dinner:

Calories	Protein	Sugar	Carbs

Wednesday

Breakfast:

Calories	Protein	Sugar	Carbs

Lunch:

Calories	Protein	Sugar	Carbs

Dinner:

Calories	Protein	Sugar	Carbs

Thursday

Breakfast:

Calories	Protein	Carbs

Lunch:

Calories	Protein	Sugar	Carbs

Dinner:

Calories	Protein	Sugar	Carbs

Friday

Breakfast:

Calories	Protein	Sugar	Carbs

Lunch:

Calories	Protein	Sugar	Carbs

Dinner:

Calories	Protein	Sugar	Carbs

Saturday

Breakfast:

Calories	Protein	Sugar	Carbs

Lunch:

Calories	Protein	Sugar	Carbs

Dinner:

Calories	Protein	Sugar	Carbs

Shopping List:

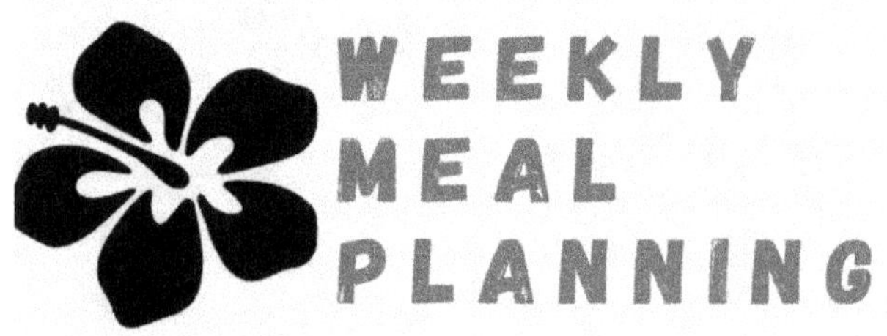

WEEKLY MEAL PLANNING

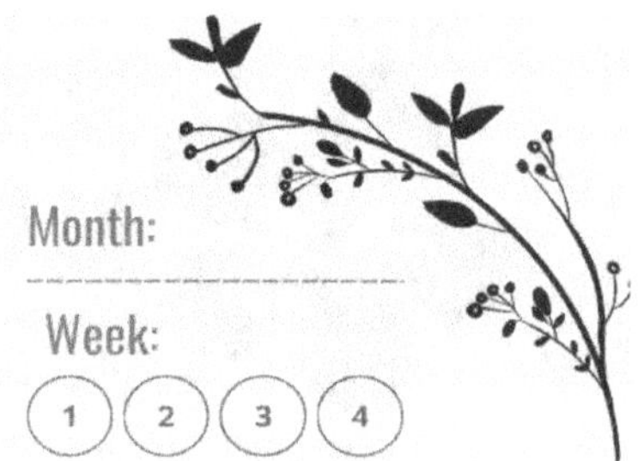

Month:

Week: 1 2 3 4

Sunday

Breakfast:

Calories	Protein	Sugar	Carbs

Lunch:

Calories	Protein	Sugar	Carbs

Dinner:

Calories	Protein	Sugar	Carbs

Monday

Breakfast:

Calories	Protein	Sugar	Carbs

Lunch:

Calories	Protein	Sugar	Carbs

Dinner:

Calories	Protein	Sugar	Carbs

Tuesday

Breakfast:

Calories	Protein	Sugar	Carbs

Lunch:

Calories	Protein	Sugar	Carbs

Dinner:

Calories	Protein	Sugar	Carbs

Wednesday

Breakfast:

Calories	Protein	Sugar	Carbs

Lunch:

Calories	Protein	Sugar	Carbs

Dinner:

Calories	Protein	Sugar	Carbs

Thursday

Breakfast:

Calories	Protein		Carbs

Lunch:

Calories	Protein	Sugar	Carbs

Dinner:

Calories	Protein	Sugar	Carbs

Friday

Breakfast:

Calories	Protein	Sugar	Carbs

Lunch:

Calories	Protein	Sugar	Carbs

Dinner:

Calories	Protein	Sugar	Carbs

Saturday

Breakfast:

Calories	Protein	Sugar	Carbs

Lunch:

Calories	Protein	Sugar	Carbs

Dinner:

Calories	Protein	Sugar	Carbs

Shopping List:

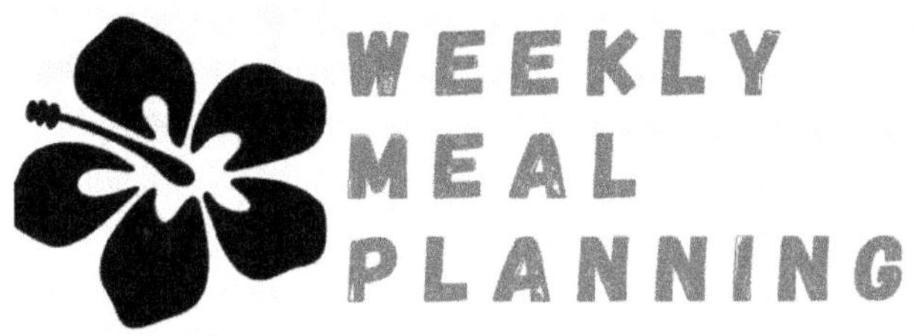

WEEKLY MEAL PLANNING

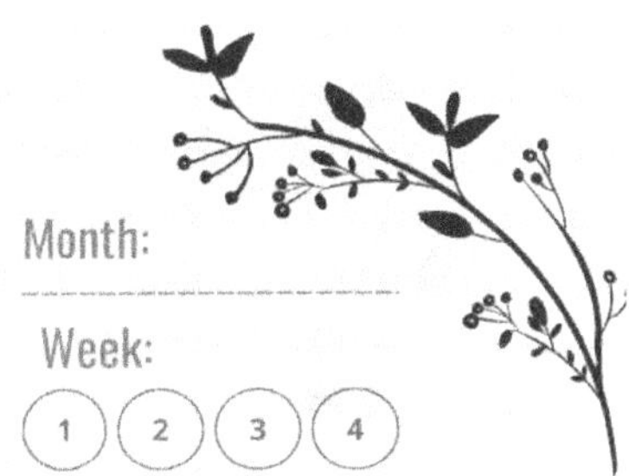

Month:

Week:

(1) (2) (3) (4)

Sunday

Breakfast:

Calories	Protein	Sugar	Carbs

Lunch:

Calories	Protein	Sugar	Carbs

Dinner:

Calories	Protein	Sugar	Carbs

Monday

Breakfast:

Calories	Protein	Sugar	Carbs

Lunch:

Calories	Protein	Sugar	Carbs

Dinner:

Calories	Protein	Sugar	Carbs

Tuesday

Breakfast:

Calories	Protein	Sugar	Carbs

Lunch:

Calories	Protein	Sugar	Carbs

Dinner:

Calories	Protein	Sugar	Carbs

Wednesday

Breakfast:

Calories	Protein	Sugar	Carbs

Lunch:

Calories	Protein	Sugar	Carbs

Dinner:

Calories	Protein	Sugar	Carbs

Thursday

Breakfast:

Calories	Protein	Carbs

Lunch:

Calories	Protein	Sugar	Carbs

Dinner:

Calories	Protein	Sugar	Carbs

Friday

Breakfast:

Calories	Protein	Sugar	Carbs

Lunch:

Calories	Protein	Sugar	Carbs

Dinner:

Calories	Protein	Sugar	Carbs

Saturday

Breakfast:

Calories	Protein	Sugar	Carbs

Lunch:

Calories	Protein	Sugar	Carbs

Dinner:

Calories	Protein	Sugar	Carbs

Shopping List:

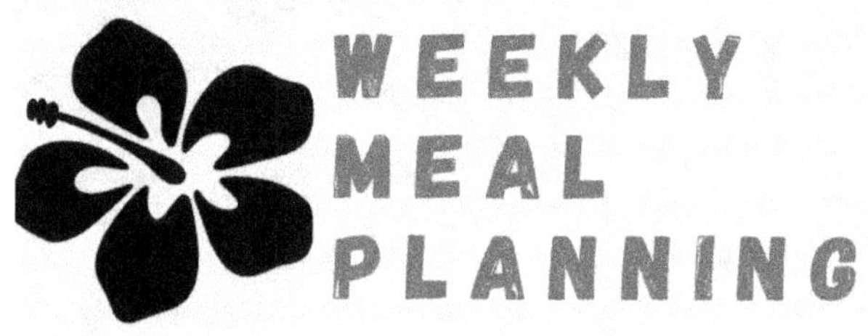

WEEKLY MEAL PLANNING

Month: _______

Week: (1) (2) (3) (4)

Sunday

Breakfast: _______

Calories	Protein	Sugar	Carbs

Lunch: _______

Calories	Protein	Sugar	Carbs

Dinner: _______

Calories	Protein	Sugar	Carbs

Monday

Breakfast: _______

Calories	Protein	Sugar	Carbs

Lunch: _______

Calories	Protein	Sugar	Carbs

Dinner: _______

Calories	Protein	Sugar	Carbs

Tuesday

Breakfast: _______

Calories	Protein	Sugar	Carbs

Lunch: _______

Calories	Protein	Sugar	Carbs

Dinner: _______

Calories	Protein	Sugar	Carbs

Wednesday

Breakfast: _______

Calories	Protein	Sugar	Carbs

Lunch: _______

Calories	Protein	Sugar	Carbs

Dinner: _______

Calories	Protein	Sugar	Carbs

Thursday

Breakfast: _______

Calories	Protein		Carbs

Lunch: _______

Calories	Protein	Sugar	Carbs

Dinner: _______

Calories	Protein	Sugar	Carbs

Friday

Breakfast: _______

Calories	Protein	Sugar	Carbs

Lunch: _______

Calories	Protein	Sugar	Carbs

Dinner: _______

Calories	Protein	Sugar	Carbs

Saturday

Breakfast: _______

Calories	Protein	Sugar	Carbs

Lunch: _______

Calories	Protein	Sugar	Carbs

Dinner: _______

Calories	Protein	Sugar	Carbs

Shopping List:

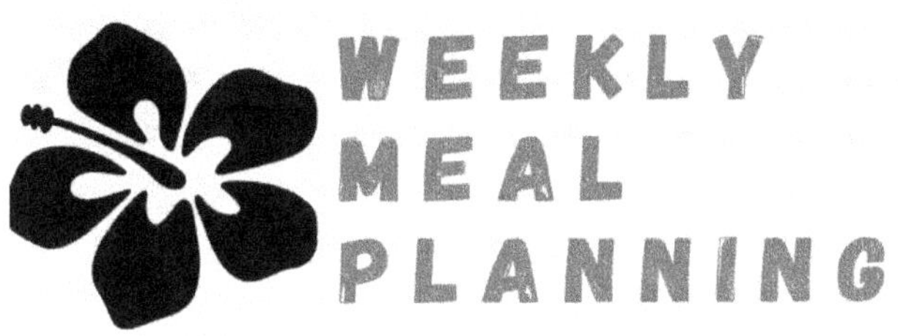

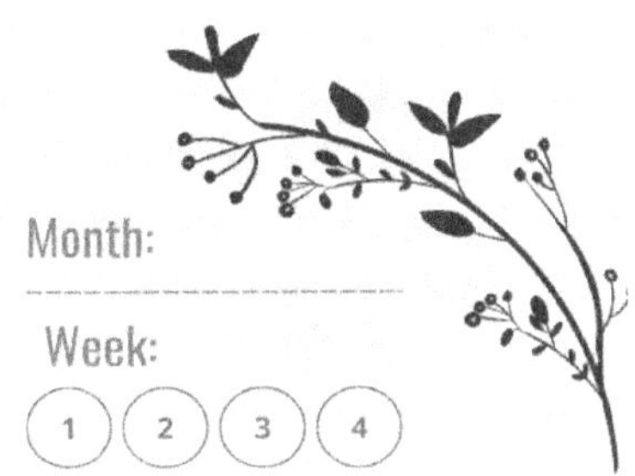

Month:

Week:
1 2 3 4

Sunday

Breakfast:
Calories Protein Sugar Carbs

Lunch:
Calories Protein Sugar Carbs

Dinner:
Calories Protein Sugar Carbs

Monday

Breakfast:
Calories Protein Sugar Carbs

Lunch:
Calories Protein Sugar Carbs

Dinner:
Calories Protein Sugar Carbs

Tuesday

Breakfast:
Calories Protein Sugar Carbs

Lunch:
Calories Protein Sugar Carbs

Dinner:
Calories Protein Sugar Carbs

Wednesday

Breakfast:
Calories Protein Sugar Carbs

Lunch:
Calories Protein Sugar Carbs

Dinner:
Calories Protein Sugar Carbs

Thursday

Breakfast:
Calories Protein Carbs

Lunch:
Calories Protein Sugar Carbs

Dinner:
Calories Protein Sugar Carbs

Friday

Breakfast:
Calories Protein Sugar Carbs

Lunch:
Calories Protein Sugar Carbs

Dinner:
Calories Protein Sugar Carbs

Saturday

Breakfast:
Calories Protein Sugar Carbs

Lunch:
Calories Protein Sugar Carbs

Dinner:
Calories Protein Sugar Carbs

Shopping List:

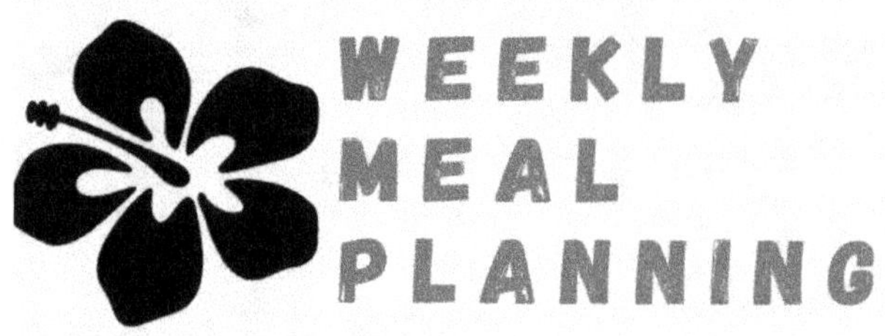

WEEKLY MEAL PLANNING

Month: ____________

Week: ① ② ③ ④

Sunday

Breakfast: ____________

Calories	Protein	Sugar	Carbs

Lunch: ____________

Calories	Protein	Sugar	Carbs

Dinner: ____________

Calories	Protein	Sugar	Carbs

Monday

Breakfast: ____________

Calories	Protein	Sugar	Carbs

Lunch: ____________

Calories	Protein	Sugar	Carbs

Dinner: ____________

Calories	Protein	Sugar	Carbs

Tuesday

Breakfast: ____________

Calories	Protein	Sugar	Carbs

Lunch: ____________

Calories	Protein	Sugar	Carbs

Dinner: ____________

Calories	Protein	Sugar	Carbs

Wednesday

Breakfast: ____________

Calories	Protein	Sugar	Carbs

Lunch: ____________

Calories	Protein	Sugar	Carbs

Dinner: ____________

Calories	Protein	Sugar	Carbs

Thursday

Breakfast: ____________

Calories	Protein		Carbs

Lunch: ____________

Calories	Protein	Sugar	Carbs

Dinner: ____________

Calories	Protein	Sugar	Carbs

Friday

Breakfast: ____________

Calories	Protein	Sugar	Carbs

Lunch: ____________

Calories	Protein	Sugar	Carbs

Dinner: ____________

Calories	Protein	Sugar	Carbs

Saturday

Breakfast: ____________

Calories	Protein	Sugar	Carbs

Lunch: ____________

Calories	Protein	Sugar	Carbs

Dinner: ____________

Calories	Protein	Sugar	Carbs

Shopping List:

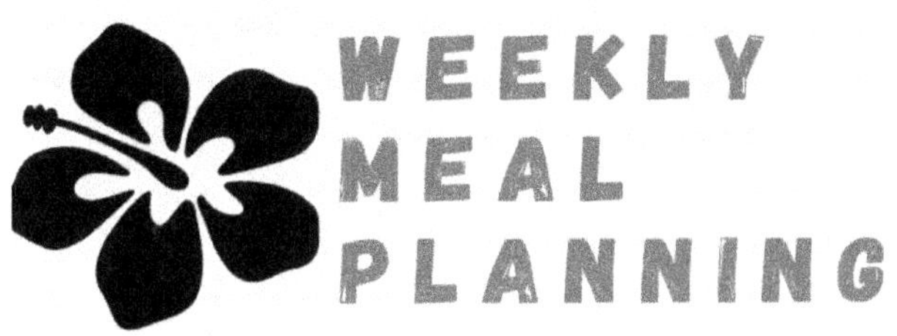

WEEKLY MEAL PLANNING

Month: _______________

Week: (1) (2) (3) (4)

Sunday

Breakfast: _______________

Calories	Protein	Sugar	Carbs

Lunch: _______________

Calories	Protein	Sugar	Carbs

Dinner: _______________

Calories	Protein	Sugar	Carbs

Monday

Breakfast: _______________

Calories	Protein	Sugar	Carbs

Lunch: _______________

Calories	Protein	Sugar	Carbs

Dinner: _______________

Calories	Protein	Sugar	Carbs

Tuesday

Breakfast: _______________

Calories	Protein	Sugar	Carbs

Lunch: _______________

Calories	Protein	Sugar	Carbs

Dinner: _______________

Calories	Protein	Sugar	Carbs

Wednesday

Breakfast: _______________

Calories	Protein	Sugar	Carbs

Lunch: _______________

Calories	Protein	Sugar	Carbs

Dinner: _______________

Calories	Protein	Sugar	Carbs

Thursday

Breakfast: _______________

Calories	Protein	Sugar	Carbs

Lunch: _______________

Calories	Protein	Sugar	Carbs

Dinner: _______________

Calories	Protein	Sugar	Carbs

Friday

Breakfast: _______________

Calories	Protein	Sugar	Carbs

Lunch: _______________

Calories	Protein	Sugar	Carbs

Dinner: _______________

Calories	Protein	Sugar	Carbs

Saturday

Breakfast: _______________

Calories	Protein	Sugar	Carbs

Lunch: _______________

Calories	Protein	Sugar	Carbs

Dinner: _______________

Calories	Protein	Sugar	Carbs

Shopping List:

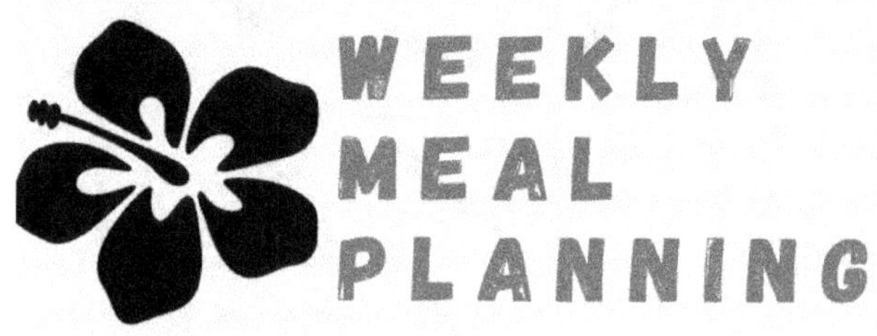

Month:

Week:

(1) (2) (3) (4)

Sunday

Breakfast:

Calories	Protein	Sugar	Carbs

Lunch:

Calories	Protein	Sugar	Carbs

Dinner:

Calories	Protein	Sugar	Carbs

Monday

Breakfast:

Calories	Protein	Sugar	Carbs

Lunch:

Calories	Protein	Sugar	Carbs

Dinner:

Calories	Protein	Sugar	Carbs

Tuesday

Breakfast:

Calories	Protein	Sugar	Carbs

Lunch:

Calories	Protein	Sugar	Carbs

Dinner:

Calories	Protein	Sugar	Carbs

Wednesday

Breakfast:

Calories	Protein	Sugar	Carbs

Lunch:

Calories	Protein	Sugar	Carbs

Dinner:

Calories	Protein	Sugar	Carbs

Thursday

Breakfast:

Calories	Protein	Sugar	Carbs

Lunch:

Calories	Protein	Sugar	Carbs

Dinner:

Calories	Protein	Sugar	Carbs

Friday

Breakfast:

Calories	Protein	Sugar	Carbs

Lunch:

Calories	Protein	Sugar	Carbs

Dinner:

Calories	Protein	Sugar	Carbs

Saturday

Breakfast:

Calories	Protein	Sugar	Carbs

Lunch:

Calories	Protein	Sugar	Carbs

Dinner:

Calories	Protein	Sugar	Carbs

Shopping List:

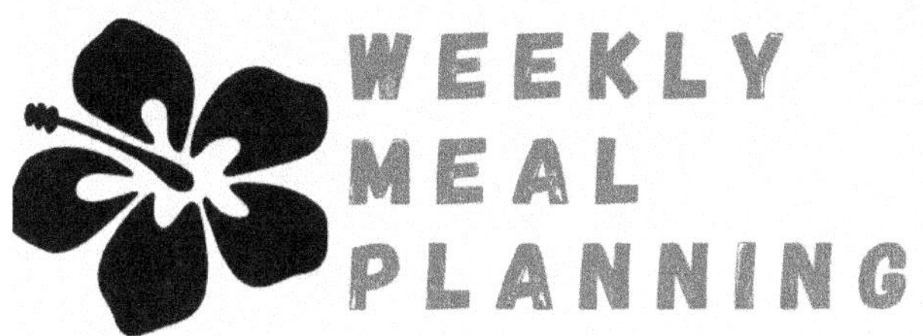

WEEKLY MEAL PLANNING

Month:

Week:

(1) (2) (3) (4)

Sunday

Breakfast:

Calories	Protein	Sugar	Carbs

Lunch:

Calories	Protein	Sugar	Carbs

Dinner:

Calories	Protein	Sugar	Carbs

Monday

Breakfast:

Calories	Protein	Sugar	Carbs

Lunch:

Calories	Protein	Sugar	Carbs

Dinner:

Calories	Protein	Sugar	Carbs

Tuesday

Breakfast:

Calories	Protein	Sugar	Carbs

Lunch:

Calories	Protein	Sugar	Carbs

Dinner:

Calories	Protein	Sugar	Carbs

Wednesday

Breakfast:

Calories	Protein	Sugar	Carbs

Lunch:

Calories	Protein	Sugar	Carbs

Dinner:

Calories	Protein	Sugar	Carbs

Thursday

Breakfast:

Calories	Protein	Carbs

Lunch:

Calories	Protein	Sugar	Carbs

Dinner:

Calories	Protein	Sugar	Carbs

Friday

Breakfast:

Calories	Protein	Sugar	Carbs

Lunch:

Calories	Protein	Sugar	Carbs

Dinner:

Calories	Protein	Sugar	Carbs

Saturday

Breakfast:

Calories	Protein	Sugar	Carbs

Lunch:

Calories	Protein	Sugar	Carbs

Dinner:

Calories	Protein	Sugar	Carbs

Shopping List:

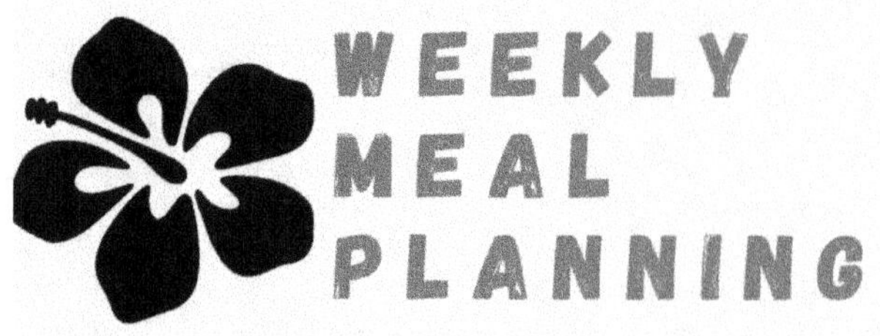

WEEKLY MEAL PLANNING

Month: ______

Week: (1) (2) (3) (4)

Sunday

Breakfast: ______

Calories	Protein	Sugar	Carbs

Lunch: ______

Calories	Protein	Sugar	Carbs

Dinner: ______

Calories	Protein	Sugar	Carbs

Monday

Breakfast: ______

Calories	Protein	Sugar	Carbs

Lunch: ______

Calories	Protein	Sugar	Carbs

Dinner: ______

Calories	Protein	Sugar	Carbs

Tuesday

Breakfast: ______

Calories	Protein	Sugar	Carbs

Lunch: ______

Calories	Protein	Sugar	Carbs

Dinner: ______

Calories	Protein	Sugar	Carbs

Wednesday

Breakfast: ______

Calories	Protein	Sugar	Carbs

Lunch: ______

Calories	Protein	Sugar	Carbs

Dinner: ______

Calories	Protein	Sugar	Carbs

Thursday

Breakfast: ______

Calories	Protein	Sugar	Carbs

Lunch: ______

Calories	Protein	Sugar	Carbs

Dinner: ______

Calories	Protein	Sugar	Carbs

Friday

Breakfast: ______

Calories	Protein	Sugar	Carbs

Lunch: ______

Calories	Protein	Sugar	Carbs

Dinner: ______

Calories	Protein	Sugar	Carbs

Saturday

Breakfast: ______

Calories	Protein	Sugar	Carbs

Lunch: ______

Calories	Protein	Sugar	Carbs

Dinner: ______

Calories	Protein	Sugar	Carbs

Shopping List:

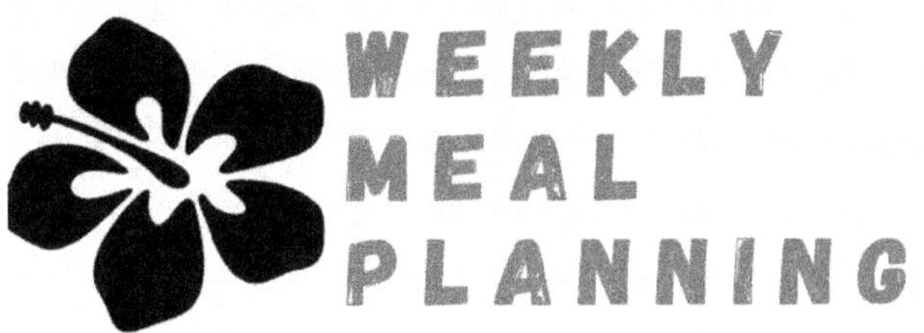

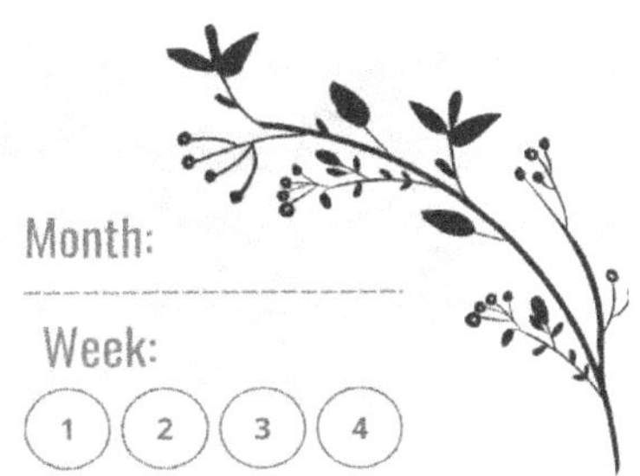

Month: _______________

Week: (1) (2) (3) (4)

Sunday

Breakfast: _______________

Calories	Protein	Sugar	Carbs

Lunch: _______________

Calories	Protein	Sugar	Carbs

Dinner: _______________

Calories	Protein	Sugar	Carbs

Monday

Breakfast: _______________

Calories	Protein	Sugar	Carbs

Lunch: _______________

Calories	Protein	Sugar	Carbs

Dinner: _______________

Calories	Protein	Sugar	Carbs

Tuesday

Breakfast: _______________

Calories	Protein	Sugar	Carbs

Lunch: _______________

Calories	Protein	Sugar	Carbs

Dinner: _______________

Calories	Protein	Sugar	Carbs

Wednesday

Breakfast: _______________

Calories	Protein	Sugar	Carbs

Lunch: _______________

Calories	Protein	Sugar	Carbs

Dinner: _______________

Calories	Protein	Sugar	Carbs

Thursday

Breakfast: _______________

Calories	Protein	Sugar	Carbs

Lunch: _______________

Calories	Protein	Sugar	Carbs

Dinner: _______________

Calories	Protein	Sugar	Carbs

Friday

Breakfast: _______________

Calories	Protein	Sugar	Carbs

Lunch: _______________

Calories	Protein	Sugar	Carbs

Dinner: _______________

Calories	Protein	Sugar	Carbs

Saturday

Breakfast: _______________

Calories	Protein	Sugar	Carbs

Lunch: _______________

Calories	Protein	Sugar	Carbs

Dinner: _______________

Calories	Protein	Sugar	Carbs

Shopping List:

____
____
____
____
____
____
____
____
____
____
____
____
____
____

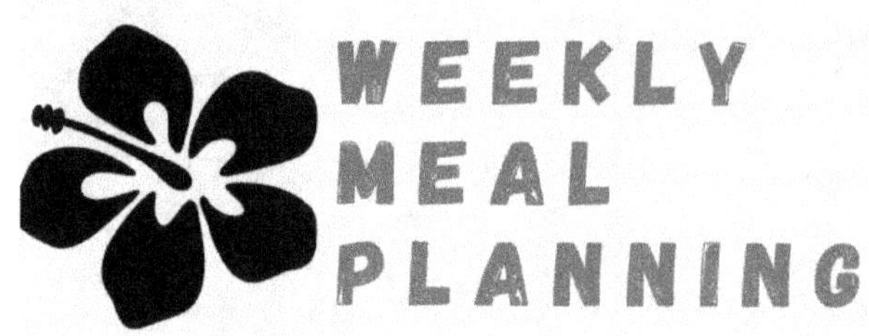

WEEKLY MEAL PLANNING

Month:

Week: 1 2 3 4

Sunday

Breakfast:

Calories	Protein	Sugar	Carbs

Lunch:

Calories	Protein	Sugar	Carbs

Dinner:

Calories	Protein	Sugar	Carbs

Monday

Breakfast:

Calories	Protein	Sugar	Carbs

Lunch:

Calories	Protein	Sugar	Carbs

Dinner:

Calories	Protein	Sugar	Carbs

Tuesday

Breakfast:

Calories	Protein	Sugar	Carbs

Lunch:

Calories	Protein	Sugar	Carbs

Dinner:

Calories	Protein	Sugar	Carbs

Wednesday

Breakfast:

Calories	Protein	Sugar	Carbs

Lunch:

Calories	Protein	Sugar	Carbs

Dinner:

Calories	Protein	Sugar	Carbs

Thursday

Breakfast:

Calories	Protein		Carbs

Lunch:

Calories	Protein	Sugar	Carbs

Dinner:

Calories	Protein	Sugar	Carbs

Friday

Breakfast:

Calories	Protein	Sugar	Carbs

Lunch:

Calories	Protein	Sugar	Carbs

Dinner:

Calories	Protein	Sugar	Carbs

Saturday

Breakfast:

Calories	Protein	Sugar	Carbs

Lunch:

Calories	Protein	Sugar	Carbs

Dinner:

Calories	Protein	Sugar	Carbs

Shopping List:

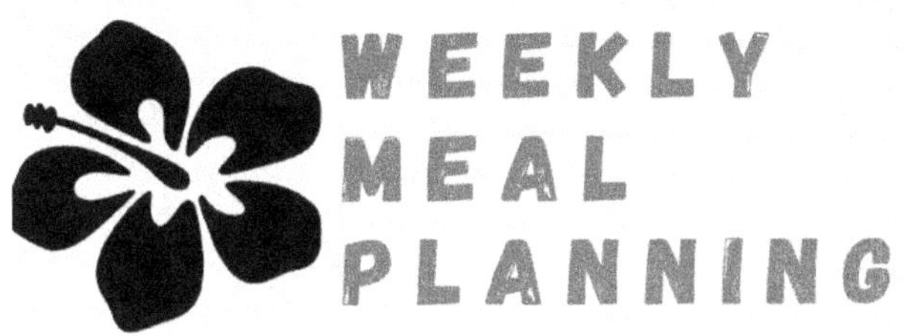

WEEKLY MEAL PLANNING

Month: _____________

Week: (1) (2) (3) (4)

Sunday

Breakfast: _____________

Calories	Protein	Sugar	Carbs

Lunch: _____________

Calories	Protein	Sugar	Carbs

Dinner: _____________

Calories	Protein	Sugar	Carbs

Monday

Breakfast: _____________

Calories	Protein	Sugar	Carbs

Lunch: _____________

Calories	Protein	Sugar	Carbs

Dinner: _____________

Calories	Protein	Sugar	Carbs

Tuesday

Breakfast: _____________

Calories	Protein	Sugar	Carbs

Lunch: _____________

Calories	Protein	Sugar	Carbs

Dinner: _____________

Calories	Protein	Sugar	Carbs

Wednesday

Breakfast: _____________

Calories	Protein	Sugar	Carbs

Lunch: _____________

Calories	Protein	Sugar	Carbs

Dinner: _____________

Calories	Protein	Sugar	Carbs

Thursday

Breakfast: _____________

Calories	Protein		Carbs

Lunch: _____________

Calories	Protein	Sugar	Carbs

Dinner: _____________

Calories	Protein	Sugar	Carbs

Friday

Breakfast: _____________

Calories	Protein	Sugar	Carbs

Lunch: _____________

Calories	Protein	Sugar	Carbs

Dinner: _____________

Calories	Protein	Sugar	Carbs

Saturday

Breakfast: _____________

Calories	Protein	Sugar	Carbs

Lunch: _____________

Calories	Protein	Sugar	Carbs

Dinner: _____________

Calories	Protein	Sugar	Carbs

Shopping List:

____

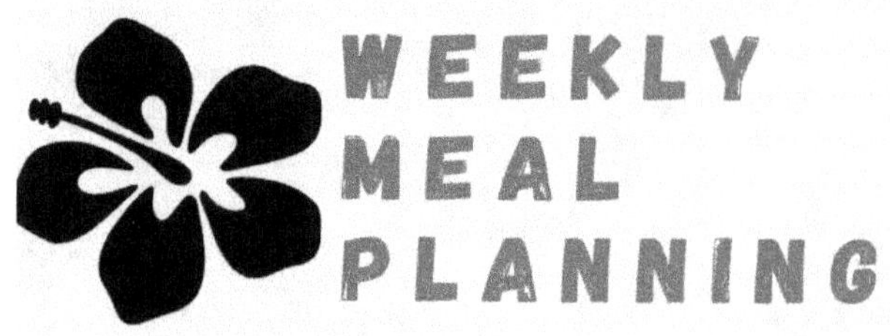

Month:

Week:
(1) (2) (3) (4)

Sunday

Breakfast:

Calories	Protein	Sugar	Carbs

Lunch:

Calories	Protein	Sugar	Carbs

Dinner:

Calories	Protein	Sugar	Carbs

Monday

Breakfast:

Calories	Protein	Sugar	Carbs

Lunch:

Calories	Protein	Sugar	Carbs

Dinner:

Calories	Protein	Sugar	Carbs

Tuesday

Breakfast:

Calories	Protein	Sugar	Carbs

Lunch:

Calories	Protein	Sugar	Carbs

Dinner:

Calories	Protein	Sugar	Carbs

Wednesday

Breakfast:

Calories	Protein	Sugar	Carbs

Lunch:

Calories	Protein	Sugar	Carbs

Dinner:

Calories	Protein	Sugar	Carbs

Thursday

Breakfast:

Calories	Protein		Carbs

Lunch:

Calories	Protein	Sugar	Carbs

Dinner:

Calories	Protein	Sugar	Carbs

Friday

Breakfast:

Calories	Protein	Sugar	Carbs

Lunch:

Calories	Protein	Sugar	Carbs

Dinner:

Calories	Protein	Sugar	Carbs

Saturday

Breakfast:

Calories	Protein	Sugar	Carbs

Lunch:

Calories	Protein	Sugar	Carbs

Dinner:

Calories	Protein	Sugar	Carbs

Shopping List:

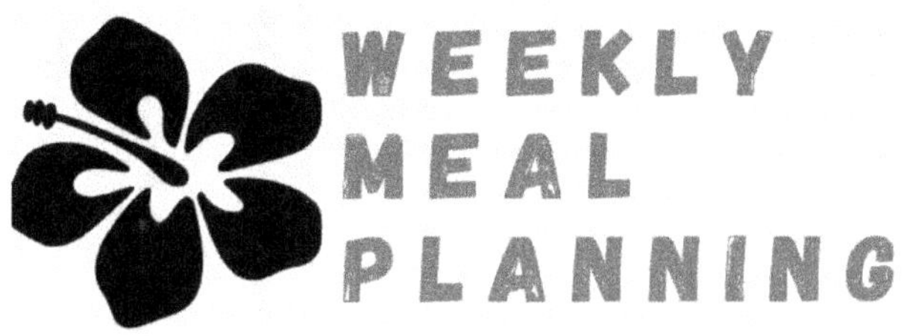

WEEKLY MEAL PLANNING

Month:

Week:
(1) (2) (3) (4)

Sunday

Breakfast:

Calories	Protein	Sugar	Carbs

Lunch:

Calories	Protein	Sugar	Carbs

Dinner:

Calories	Protein	Sugar	Carbs

Monday

Breakfast:

Calories	Protein	Sugar	Carbs

Lunch:

Calories	Protein	Sugar	Carbs

Dinner:

Calories	Protein	Sugar	Carbs

Tuesday

Breakfast:

Calories	Protein	Sugar	Carbs

Lunch:

Calories	Protein	Sugar	Carbs

Dinner:

Calories	Protein	Sugar	Carbs

Wednesday

Breakfast:

Calories	Protein	Sugar	Carbs

Lunch:

Calories	Protein	Sugar	Carbs

Dinner:

Calories	Protein	Sugar	Carbs

Thursday

Breakfast:

Calories	Protein	Carbs

Lunch:

Calories	Protein	Sugar	Carbs

Dinner:

Calories	Protein	Sugar	Carbs

Friday

Breakfast:

Calories	Protein	Sugar	Carbs

Lunch:

Calories	Protein	Sugar	Carbs

Dinner:

Calories	Protein	Sugar	Carbs

Saturday

Breakfast:

Calories	Protein	Sugar	Carbs

Lunch:

Calories	Protein	Sugar	Carbs

Dinner:

Calories	Protein	Sugar	Carbs

Shopping List:

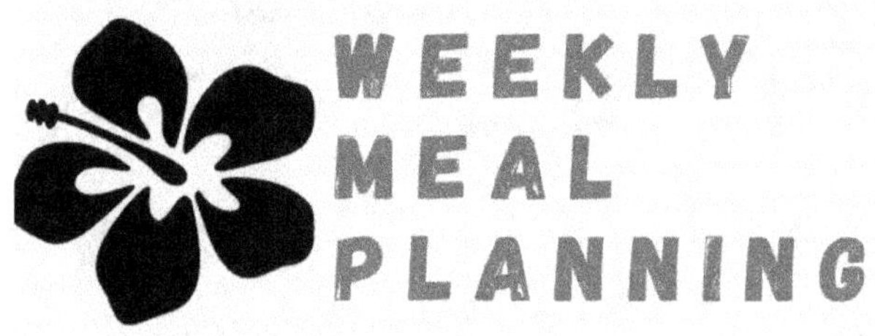

Month:

Week:
(1) (2) (3) (4)

Sunday

Breakfast:

Calories	Protein	Sugar	Carbs

Lunch:

Calories	Protein	Sugar	Carbs

Dinner:

Calories	Protein	Sugar	Carbs

Monday

Breakfast:

Calories	Protein	Sugar	Carbs

Lunch:

Calories	Protein	Sugar	Carbs

Dinner:

Calories	Protein	Sugar	Carbs

Tuesday

Breakfast:

Calories	Protein	Sugar	Carbs

Lunch:

Calories	Protein	Sugar	Carbs

Dinner:

Calories	Protein	Sugar	Carbs

Wednesday

Breakfast:

Calories	Protein	Sugar	Carbs

Lunch:

Calories	Protein	Sugar	Carbs

Dinner:

Calories	Protein	Sugar	Carbs

Thursday

Breakfast:

Calories	Protein	Carbs

Lunch:

Calories	Protein	Sugar	Carbs

Dinner:

Calories	Protein	Sugar	Carbs

Friday

Breakfast:

Calories	Protein	Sugar	Carbs

Lunch:

Calories	Protein	Sugar	Carbs

Dinner:

Calories	Protein	Sugar	Carbs

Saturday

Breakfast:

Calories	Protein	Sugar	Carbs

Lunch:

Calories	Protein	Sugar	Carbs

Dinner:

Calories	Protein	Sugar	Carbs

Shopping List:

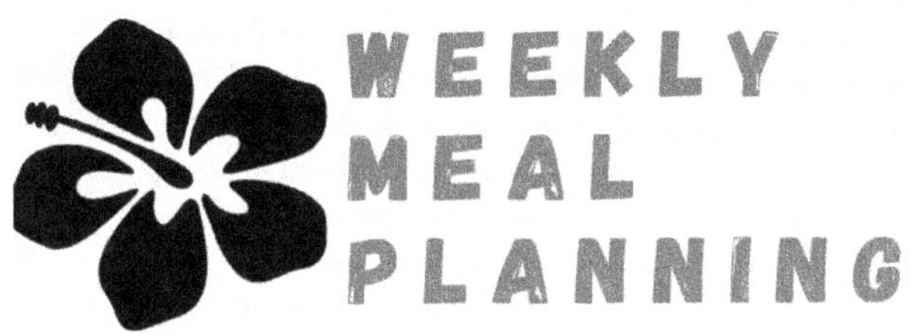

WEEKLY MEAL PLANNING

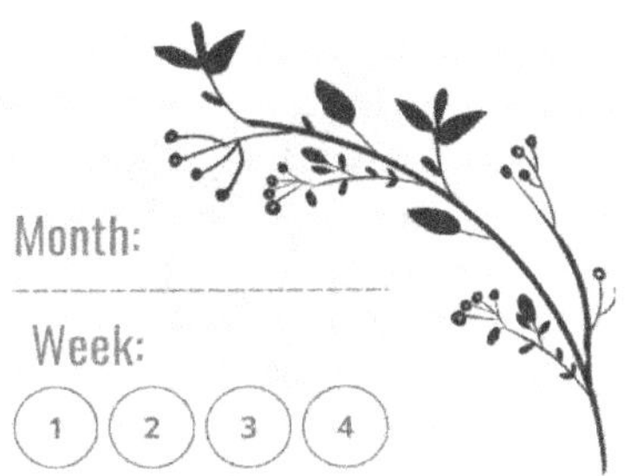

Month:

Week:
(1) (2) (3) (4)

Sunday

Breakfast:

Calories	Protein	Sugar	Carbs

Lunch:

Calories	Protein	Sugar	Carbs

Dinner:

Calories	Protein	Sugar	Carbs

Monday

Breakfast:

Calories	Protein	Sugar	Carbs

Lunch:

Calories	Protein	Sugar	Carbs

Dinner:

Calories	Protein	Sugar	Carbs

Tuesday

Breakfast:

Calories	Protein	Sugar	Carbs

Lunch:

Calories	Protein	Sugar	Carbs

Dinner:

Calories	Protein	Sugar	Carbs

Wednesday

Breakfast:

Calories	Protein	Sugar	Carbs

Lunch:

Calories	Protein	Sugar	Carbs

Dinner:

Calories	Protein	Sugar	Carbs

Thursday

Breakfast:

Calories	Protein	Carbs

Lunch:

Calories	Protein	Sugar	Carbs

Dinner:

Calories	Protein	Sugar	Carbs

Friday

Breakfast:

Calories	Protein	Sugar	Carbs

Lunch:

Calories	Protein	Sugar	Carbs

Dinner:

Calories	Protein	Sugar	Carbs

Saturday

Breakfast:

Calories	Protein	Sugar	Carbs

Lunch:

Calories	Protein	Sugar	Carbs

Dinner:

Calories	Protein	Sugar	Carbs

Shopping List:

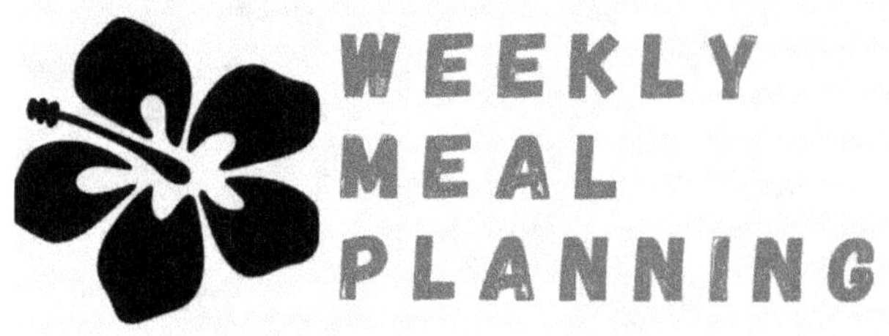

Month:

Week:

(1) (2) (3) (4)

Sunday

Breakfast:

Calories	Protein	Sugar	Carbs

Lunch:

Calories	Protein	Sugar	Carbs

Dinner:

Calories	Protein	Sugar	Carbs

Monday

Breakfast:

Calories	Protein	Sugar	Carbs

Lunch:

Calories	Protein	Sugar	Carbs

Dinner:

Calories	Protein	Sugar	Carbs

Tuesday

Breakfast:

Calories	Protein	Sugar	Carbs

Lunch:

Calories	Protein	Sugar	Carbs

Dinner:

Calories	Protein	Sugar	Carbs

Wednesday

Breakfast:

Calories	Protein	Sugar	Carbs

Lunch:

Calories	Protein	Sugar	Carbs

Dinner:

Calories	Protein	Sugar	Carbs

Thursday

Breakfast:

Calories	Protein	Carbs

Lunch:

Calories	Protein	Sugar	Carbs

Dinner:

Calories	Protein	Sugar	Carbs

Friday

Breakfast:

Calories	Protein	Sugar	Carbs

Lunch:

Calories	Protein	Sugar	Carbs

Dinner:

Calories	Protein	Sugar	Carbs

Saturday

Breakfast:

Calories	Protein	Sugar	Carbs

Lunch:

Calories	Protein	Sugar	Carbs

Dinner:

Calories	Protein	Sugar	Carbs

Shopping List:

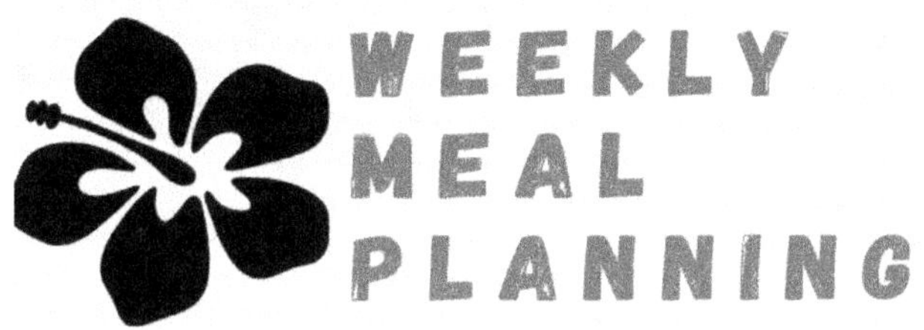

WEEKLY MEAL PLANNING

Month: ______________

Week: ① ② ③ ④

Sunday

Breakfast: ______________

Calories	Protein	Sugar	Carbs

Lunch: ______________

Calories	Protein	Sugar	Carbs

Dinner: ______________

Calories	Protein	Sugar	Carbs

Monday

Breakfast: ______________

Calories	Protein	Sugar	Carbs

Lunch: ______________

Calories	Protein	Sugar	Carbs

Dinner: ______________

Calories	Protein	Sugar	Carbs

Tuesday

Breakfast: ______________

Calories	Protein	Sugar	Carbs

Lunch: ______________

Calories	Protein	Sugar	Carbs

Dinner: ______________

Calories	Protein	Sugar	Carbs

Wednesday

Breakfast: ______________

Calories	Protein	Sugar	Carbs

Lunch: ______________

Calories	Protein	Sugar	Carbs

Dinner: ______________

Calories	Protein	Sugar	Carbs

Thursday

Breakfast: ______________

Calories	Protein	Carbs

Lunch: ______________

Calories	Protein	Sugar	Carbs

Dinner: ______________

Calories	Protein	Sugar	Carbs

Friday

Breakfast: ______________

Calories	Protein	Sugar	Carbs

Lunch: ______________

Calories	Protein	Sugar	Carbs

Dinner: ______________

Calories	Protein	Sugar	Carbs

Saturday

Breakfast: ______________

Calories	Protein	Sugar	Carbs

Lunch: ______________

Calories	Protein	Sugar	Carbs

Dinner: ______________

Calories	Protein	Sugar	Carbs

Shopping List:

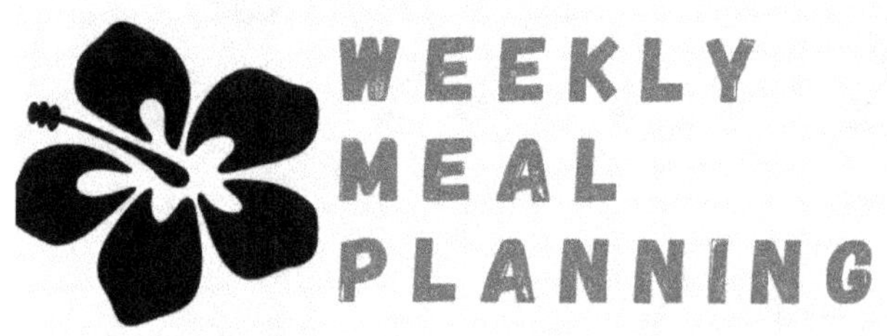

Month:

Week:

1 2 3 4

Sunday

Breakfast:

Calories	Protein	Sugar	Carbs

Lunch:

Calories	Protein	Sugar	Carbs

Dinner:

Calories	Protein	Sugar	Carbs

Monday

Breakfast:

Calories	Protein	Sugar	Carbs

Lunch:

Calories	Protein	Sugar	Carbs

Dinner:

Calories	Protein	Sugar	Carbs

Tuesday

Breakfast:

Calories	Protein	Sugar	Carbs

Lunch:

Calories	Protein	Sugar	Carbs

Dinner:

Calories	Protein	Sugar	Carbs

Wednesday

Breakfast:

Calories	Protein	Sugar	Carbs

Lunch:

Calories	Protein	Sugar	Carbs

Dinner:

Calories	Protein	Sugar	Carbs

Thursday

Breakfast:

Calories	Protein		Carbs

Lunch:

Calories	Protein	Sugar	Carbs

Dinner:

Calories	Protein	Sugar	Carbs

Friday

Breakfast:

Calories	Protein	Sugar	Carbs

Lunch:

Calories	Protein	Sugar	Carbs

Dinner:

Calories	Protein	Sugar	Carbs

Saturday

Breakfast:

Calories	Protein	Sugar	Carbs

Lunch:

Calories	Protein	Sugar	Carbs

Dinner:

Calories	Protein	Sugar	Carbs

Shopping List:

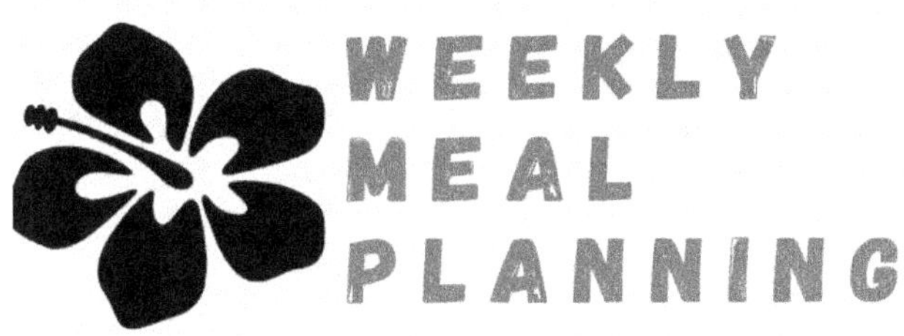

WEEKLY MEAL PLANNING

Month: _______________

Week:

(1) (2) (3) (4)

Sunday

Breakfast: _______________

Calories	Protein	Sugar	Carbs

Lunch: _______________

Calories	Protein	Sugar	Carbs

Dinner: _______________

Calories	Protein	Sugar	Carbs

Monday

Breakfast: _______________

Calories	Protein	Sugar	Carbs

Lunch: _______________

Calories	Protein	Sugar	Carbs

Dinner: _______________

Calories	Protein	Sugar	Carbs

Tuesday

Breakfast: _______________

Calories	Protein	Sugar	Carbs

Lunch: _______________

Calories	Protein	Sugar	Carbs

Dinner: _______________

Calories	Protein	Sugar	Carbs

Wednesday

Breakfast: _______________

Calories	Protein	Sugar	Carbs

Lunch: _______________

Calories	Protein	Sugar	Carbs

Dinner: _______________

Calories	Protein	Sugar	Carbs

Thursday

Breakfast: _______________

Calories	Protein	Carbs

Lunch: _______________

Calories	Protein	Sugar	Carbs

Dinner: _______________

Calories	Protein	Sugar	Carbs

Friday

Breakfast: _______________

Calories	Protein	Sugar	Carbs

Lunch: _______________

Calories	Protein	Sugar	Carbs

Dinner: _______________

Calories	Protein	Sugar	Carbs

Saturday

Breakfast: _______________

Calories	Protein	Sugar	Carbs

Lunch: _______________

Calories	Protein	Sugar	Carbs

Dinner: _______________

Calories	Protein	Sugar	Carbs

Shopping List:

____
____
____
____
____
____
____
____
____
____
____
____
____

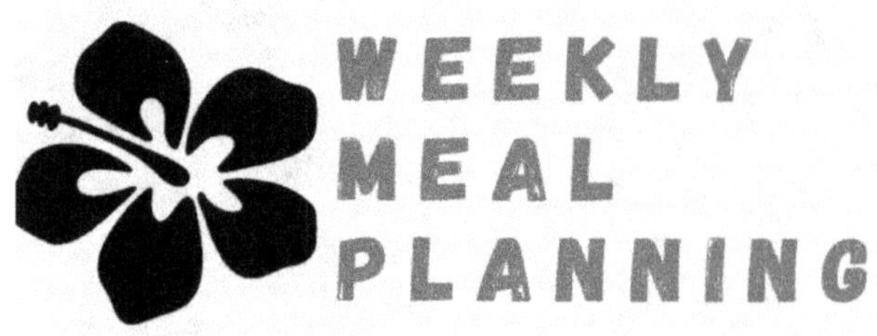

WEEKLY MEAL PLANNING

Month:

Week:
(1) (2) (3) (4)

Sunday

Breakfast:
Calories	Protein	Sugar	Carbs

Lunch:
Calories	Protein	Sugar	Carbs

Dinner:
Calories	Protein	Sugar	Carbs

Monday

Breakfast:
Calories	Protein	Sugar	Carbs

Lunch:
Calories	Protein	Sugar	Carbs

Dinner:
Calories	Protein	Sugar	Carbs

Tuesday

Breakfast:
Calories	Protein	Sugar	Carbs

Lunch:
Calories	Protein	Sugar	Carbs

Dinner:
Calories	Protein	Sugar	Carbs

Wednesday

Breakfast:
Calories	Protein	Sugar	Carbs

Lunch:
Calories	Protein	Sugar	Carbs

Dinner:
Calories	Protein	Sugar	Carbs

Thursday

Breakfast:
Calories	Protein		Carbs

Lunch:
Calories	Protein	Sugar	Carbs

Dinner:
Calories	Protein	Sugar	Carbs

Friday

Breakfast:
Calories	Protein	Sugar	Carbs

Lunch:
Calories	Protein	Sugar	Carbs

Dinner:
Calories	Protein	Sugar	Carbs

Saturday

Breakfast:
Calories	Protein	Sugar	Carbs

Lunch:
Calories	Protein	Sugar	Carbs

Dinner:
Calories	Protein	Sugar	Carbs

Shopping List:

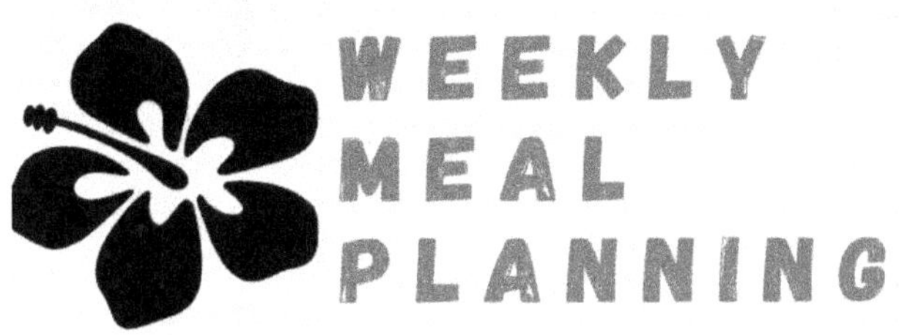

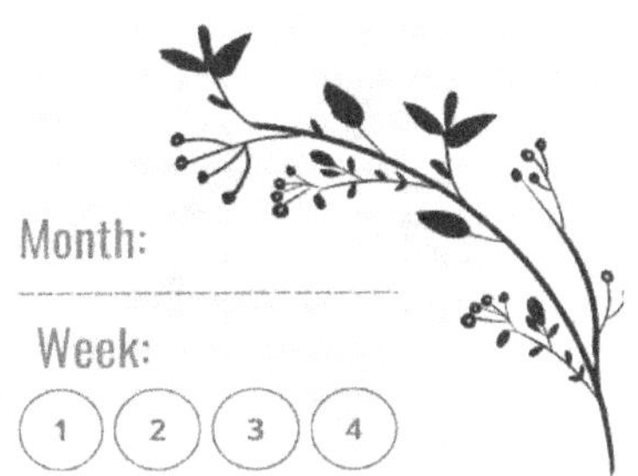

Month:

Week:
(1) (2) (3) (4)

Sunday

Breakfast:

Calories	Protein	Sugar	Carbs

Lunch:

Calories	Protein	Sugar	Carbs

Dinner:

Calories	Protein	Sugar	Carbs

Monday

Breakfast:

Calories	Protein	Sugar	Carbs

Lunch:

Calories	Protein	Sugar	Carbs

Dinner:

Calories	Protein	Sugar	Carbs

Tuesday

Breakfast:

Calories	Protein	Sugar	Carbs

Lunch:

Calories	Protein	Sugar	Carbs

Dinner:

Calories	Protein	Sugar	Carbs

Wednesday

Breakfast:

Calories	Protein	Sugar	Carbs

Lunch:

Calories	Protein	Sugar	Carbs

Dinner:

Calories	Protein	Sugar	Carbs

Thursday

Breakfast:

Calories	Protein	Carbs

Lunch:

Calories	Protein	Sugar	Carbs

Dinner:

Calories	Protein	Sugar	Carbs

Friday

Breakfast:

Calories	Protein	Sugar	Carbs

Lunch:

Calories	Protein	Sugar	Carbs

Dinner:

Calories	Protein	Sugar	Carbs

Saturday

Breakfast:

Calories	Protein	Sugar	Carbs

Lunch:

Calories	Protein	Sugar	Carbs

Dinner:

Calories	Protein	Sugar	Carbs

Shopping List:

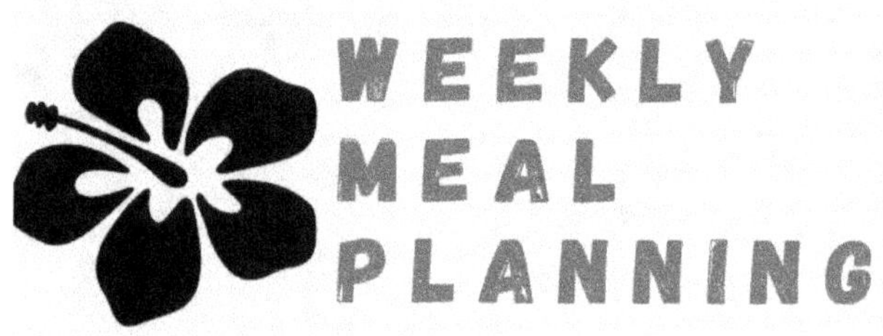

WEEKLY MEAL PLANNING

Month: _______________

Week: (1) (2) (3) (4)

Sunday

Breakfast: _______________

Calories	Protein	Sugar	Carbs

Lunch: _______________

Calories	Protein	Sugar	Carbs

Dinner: _______________

Calories	Protein	Sugar	Carbs

Monday

Breakfast: _______________

Calories	Protein	Sugar	Carbs

Lunch: _______________

Calories	Protein	Sugar	Carbs

Dinner: _______________

Calories	Protein	Sugar	Carbs

Tuesday

Breakfast: _______________

Calories	Protein	Sugar	Carbs

Lunch: _______________

Calories	Protein	Sugar	Carbs

Dinner: _______________

Calories	Protein	Sugar	Carbs

Wednesday

Breakfast: _______________

Calories	Protein	Sugar	Carbs

Lunch: _______________

Calories	Protein	Sugar	Carbs

Dinner: _______________

Calories	Protein	Sugar	Carbs

Thursday

Breakfast: _______________

Calories	Protein	Sugar	Carbs

Lunch: _______________

Calories	Protein	Sugar	Carbs

Dinner: _______________

Calories	Protein	Sugar	Carbs

Friday

Breakfast: _______________

Calories	Protein	Sugar	Carbs

Lunch: _______________

Calories	Protein	Sugar	Carbs

Dinner: _______________

Calories	Protein	Sugar	Carbs

Saturday

Breakfast: _______________

Calories	Protein	Sugar	Carbs

Lunch: _______________

Calories	Protein	Sugar	Carbs

Dinner: _______________

Calories	Protein	Sugar	Carbs

Shopping List:

____
____
____
____
____
____
____
____
____
____
____
____
____
____
____

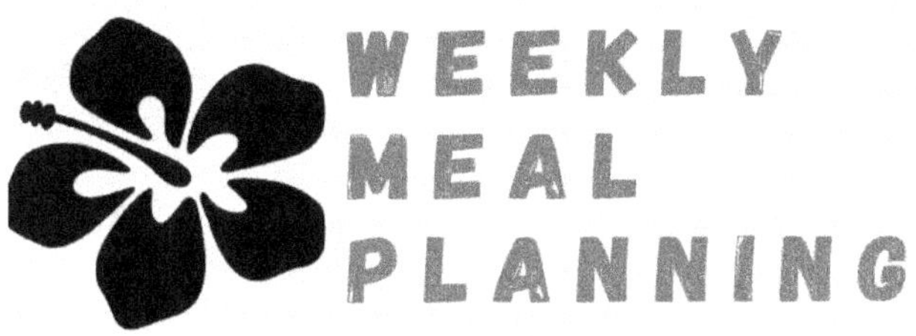

Month:

Week:
1 2 3 4

Sunday

Breakfast:
Calories	Protein	Sugar	Carbs

Lunch:
Calories	Protein	Sugar	Carbs

Dinner:
Calories	Protein	Sugar	Carbs

Monday

Breakfast:
Calories	Protein	Sugar	Carbs

Lunch:
Calories	Protein	Sugar	Carbs

Dinner:
Calories	Protein	Sugar	Carbs

Tuesday

Breakfast:
Calories	Protein	Sugar	Carbs

Lunch:
Calories	Protein	Sugar	Carbs

Dinner:
Calories	Protein	Sugar	Carbs

Wednesday

Breakfast:
Calories	Protein	Sugar	Carbs

Lunch:
Calories	Protein	Sugar	Carbs

Dinner:
Calories	Protein	Sugar	Carbs

Thursday

Breakfast:
Calories	Protein	Carbs

Lunch:
Calories	Protein	Sugar	Carbs

Dinner:
Calories	Protein	Sugar	Carbs

Friday

Breakfast:
Calories	Protein	Sugar	Carbs

Lunch:
Calories	Protein	Sugar	Carbs

Dinner:
Calories	Protein	Sugar	Carbs

Saturday

Breakfast:
Calories	Protein	Sugar	Carbs

Lunch:
Calories	Protein	Sugar	Carbs

Dinner:
Calories	Protein	Sugar	Carbs

Shopping List:

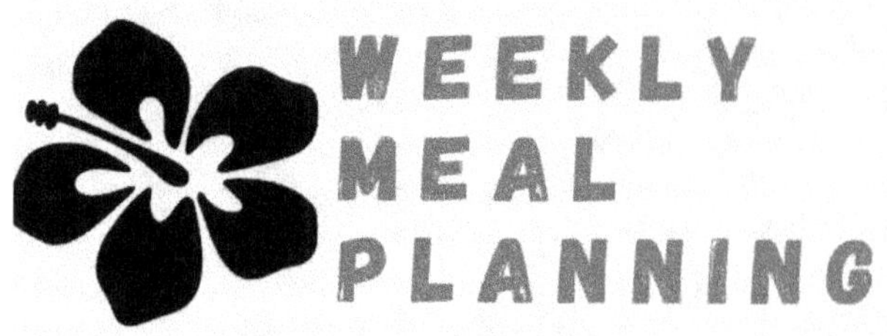

Month:

Week:
(1) (2) (3) (4)

Sunday

Breakfast:

Calories	Protein	Sugar	Carbs

Lunch:

Calories	Protein	Sugar	Carbs

Dinner:

Calories	Protein	Sugar	Carbs

Monday

Breakfast:

Calories	Protein	Sugar	Carbs

Lunch:

Calories	Protein	Sugar	Carbs

Dinner:

Calories	Protein	Sugar	Carbs

Tuesday

Breakfast:

Calories	Protein	Sugar	Carbs

Lunch:

Calories	Protein	Sugar	Carbs

Dinner:

Calories	Protein	Sugar	Carbs

Wednesday

Breakfast:

Calories	Protein	Sugar	Carbs

Lunch:

Calories	Protein	Sugar	Carbs

Dinner:

Calories	Protein	Sugar	Carbs

Thursday

Breakfast:

Calories	Protein	Carbs

Lunch:

Calories	Protein	Sugar	Carbs

Dinner:

Calories	Protein	Sugar	Carbs

Friday

Breakfast:

Calories	Protein	Sugar	Carbs

Lunch:

Calories	Protein	Sugar	Carbs

Dinner:

Calories	Protein	Sugar	Carbs

Saturday

Breakfast:

Calories	Protein	Sugar	Carbs

Lunch:

Calories	Protein	Sugar	Carbs

Dinner:

Calories	Protein	Sugar	Carbs

Shopping List:

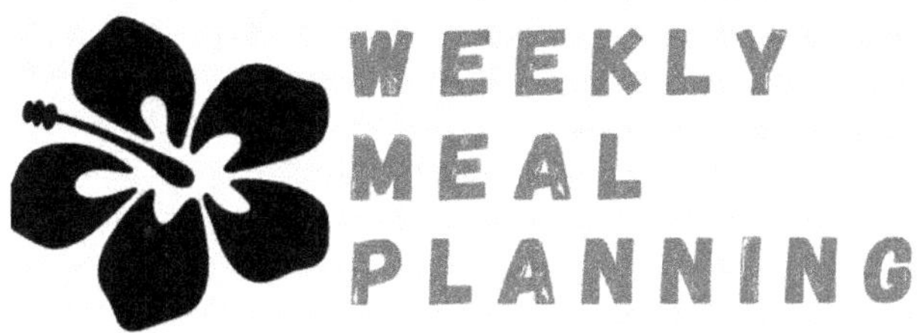

WEEKLY MEAL PLANNING

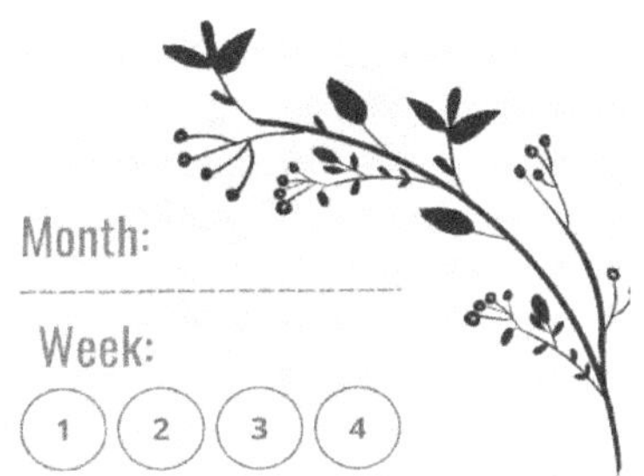

Month: _______________

Week: (1) (2) (3) (4)

Sunday

Breakfast: _______________

Calories	Protein	Sugar	Carbs

Lunch: _______________

Calories	Protein	Sugar	Carbs

Dinner: _______________

Calories	Protein	Sugar	Carbs

Monday

Breakfast: _______________

Calories	Protein	Sugar	Carbs

Lunch: _______________

Calories	Protein	Sugar	Carbs

Dinner: _______________

Calories	Protein	Sugar	Carbs

Tuesday

Breakfast: _______________

Calories	Protein	Sugar	Carbs

Lunch: _______________

Calories	Protein	Sugar	Carbs

Dinner: _______________

Calories	Protein	Sugar	Carbs

Wednesday

Breakfast: _______________

Calories	Protein	Sugar	Carbs

Lunch: _______________

Calories	Protein	Sugar	Carbs

Dinner: _______________

Calories	Protein	Sugar	Carbs

Thursday

Breakfast: _______________

Calories	Protein	Sugar	Carbs

Lunch: _______________

Calories	Protein	Sugar	Carbs

Dinner: _______________

Calories	Protein	Sugar	Carbs

Friday

Breakfast: _______________

Calories	Protein	Sugar	Carbs

Lunch: _______________

Calories	Protein	Sugar	Carbs

Dinner: _______________

Calories	Protein	Sugar	Carbs

Saturday

Breakfast: _______________

Calories	Protein	Sugar	Carbs

Lunch: _______________

Calories	Protein	Sugar	Carbs

Dinner: _______________

Calories	Protein	Sugar	Carbs

Shopping List:

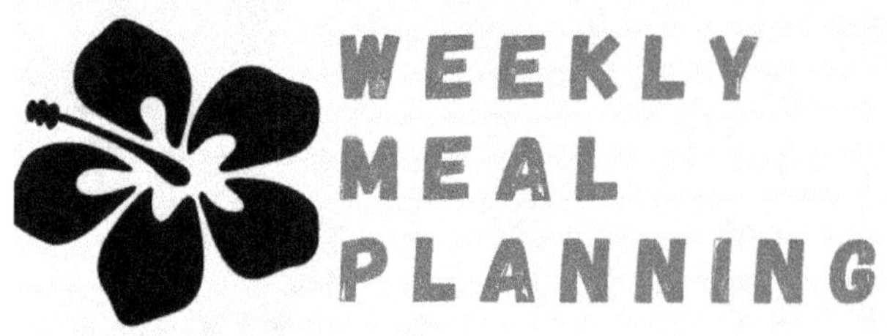

Month:

Week:
(1) (2) (3) (4)

Sunday

Breakfast:

Calories	Protein	Sugar	Carbs

Lunch:

Calories	Protein	Sugar	Carbs

Dinner:

Calories	Protein	Sugar	Carbs

Monday

Breakfast:

Calories	Protein	Sugar	Carbs

Lunch:

Calories	Protein	Sugar	Carbs

Dinner:

Calories	Protein	Sugar	Carbs

Tuesday

Breakfast:

Calories	Protein	Sugar	Carbs

Lunch:

Calories	Protein	Sugar	Carbs

Dinner:

Calories	Protein	Sugar	Carbs

Wednesday

Breakfast:

Calories	Protein	Sugar	Carbs

Lunch:

Calories	Protein	Sugar	Carbs

Dinner:

Calories	Protein	Sugar	Carbs

Thursday

Breakfast:

Calories	Protein		Carbs

Lunch:

Calories	Protein	Sugar	Carbs

Dinner:

Calories	Protein	Sugar	Carbs

Friday

Breakfast:

Calories	Protein	Sugar	Carbs

Lunch:

Calories	Protein	Sugar	Carbs

Dinner:

Calories	Protein	Sugar	Carbs

Saturday

Breakfast:

Calories	Protein	Sugar	Carbs

Lunch:

Calories	Protein	Sugar	Carbs

Dinner:

Calories	Protein	Sugar	Carbs

Shopping List: